T0149344

THE
PATIENT
ADVOCATE
HANDBOOK

How to Find and Use Your
Voice in Health Care

Liz Crocker and Claire Crocker

BALBOA.
PRESS

A DIVISION OF HAY HOUSE

The information, ideas, and suggestions in this book are not intended to render legal advice. Before following any suggestions contained in this book, you should consult your personal attorney. Neither the author nor the publisher shall be liable or responsible for any loss or damage allegedly arising as a consequence of your use or application of any information or suggestions in this book.

Balboa Press books may be ordered through booksellers or by contacting:

Balboa Press
A Division of Hay House
1663 Liberty Drive
Bloomington, IN 47403
www.balboapress.com.au
1 (877) 407-4847

Because of the dynamic nature of the Internet, any web addresses or links contained in this book may have changed since publication and may no longer be valid. The views expressed in this work are solely those of the author and do not necessarily reflect the views of the publisher, and the publisher hereby disclaims any responsibility for them.

The author of this book does not dispense medical advice or prescribe the use of any technique as a form of treatment for physical, emotional, or medical problems without the advice of a physician, either directly or indirectly. The intent of the author is only to offer information of a general nature to help you in your quest for emotional and spiritual well-being. In the event you use any of the information in this book for yourself, which is your constitutional right, the author and the publisher assume no responsibility for your actions.

Any people depicted in stock imagery provided by Getty Images are models, and such images are being used for illustrative purposes only. Certain stock imagery © Getty Images.

Print information available on the last page.

ISBN: 978-1-5043-1869-3 (sc)
ISBN: 978-1-5043-1870-9 (e)

Balboa Press rev. date: 08/06/2019

For Joan

CONTENTS

PREFACE

If you have chosen to read this Handbook, then it is likely that either you or someone you care about is currently experiencing a health challenge. For those of us who take comfort in a sense of control over our lives, nothing shakes us to our core more than the shock and vulnerability created through ill health.

Since 1973, I have practiced as a health psychologist, registered with the Australian Psychological Society, specialising in cancer and women's health. My practice is well known in Melbourne, Australia and I have long-standing relationships with many medical and health personnel and organisations.

During my career, I have actively assisted patients who have difficulty navigating their way through the health system. I have also provided regular support to many health professionals as they struggle with the ever-increasing stresses of their daily workload. These are people who went into nursing and the health field wanting to care for people and make a difference, but too often they find themselves confronted by the reality of what can actually be done for patients with the resources available.

In 2010 my family had a very stressful experience when a close relative became seriously ill. My daughter, Claire, was supporting them as they started to ricochet from one medical event to the next with astonishing speed and severity. Claire had only recently left her legal firm where she had developed a practice in family law, so she was well equipped to handle crisis and urgency. But nothing had prepared her for the sense of disempowerment she felt as she sat by the bedside of someone she loved while they endured one battle after another.

I remember when she called me after an especially difficult day. She had arrived at the hospital only to find, with no notice or warning, that urgent surgery had been scheduled for her relative that would have irreversible consequences. Her relative had been too frightened to ask any questions – they signed the consent form and the surgery took place a short time later.

When we were able to discuss and share the experience, she told me that she had stood in the corridor unable to speak (because she did not know the words), unable to act (because she did not know her rights) and unable to think (because the horror of the moment overwhelmed her). She thought: *"if I am a skilled lawyer and I feel like this, then how must so many others feel?"* She could not fault the intentions or care of the health care workers - they were immensely kind and concerned for everyone. It was no one person's fault, and yet adverse outcomes were occurring and repeating.

Claire hadn't realised at the time that she was dealing with a health system that in many ways is like a machine. It has a momentum all of its own that can sweep everyone in its wake. Even the nursing and medical staff can be swept along to find themselves operating in ways that may not fit their values, but they feel unable to change course.

After the trauma of this event, we discussed ways to help others caught in similar situations to feel that they had a voice and could be heard. We both felt there was a real opportunity to guide and support others who may experience the same feelings of disempowerment, fear, overwhelm and confusion during a health challenge. By combining my experience as a psychologist with Claire's legal and crisis management skills, the initial blueprint for the Handbook you are now reading was formed.

Between 2011 and 2016, I worked with Claire and my husband, Leigh, as private patient advocates helping many patients and their families to find their voice and to navigate their way through the health system. We established the Patient Advocate Institute and I was primarily responsible for managing a small team of volunteers. Together, we successfully supported people interested in this area to develop their confidence and skills. This Handbook is a modified version of the Training Course that was developed during that period.

As volunteers, we juggled this work with our 'day jobs'. As demand for trainings and advice grew, we realised that we lacked the resources to properly develop patient advocacy as an industry due to the other responsibilities we had with our careers and families. In 2016 we scaled back the trainings, and since then no further formal work has been undertaken by us in this field.

Then, last year, I had a near fatal health incident. Leigh was able to draw on his previous advocacy experience to help me through my own crisis so I could regain my health and make a full recovery. This event triggered within me a deep realisation that our work in patient advocacy was still very relevant, and so we decided to convert our Training Course into a new format (this Handbook) so it could be easily available and accessible to others who may also need support of this kind.

This Handbook contains everything we have learned, tested and experienced to help you to successfully manage your way through a health challenge. There is nothing contained in these pages that we have not applied ourselves. It is practical and proven. By working through this Handbook you will also be able to avoid some common pitfalls and mistakes that we have had to learn the hard way!

It is my hope that this Handbook will be a compass to help you chart a clear path forward for yourself and for those you love while you progress through the health system. I hope that it will provide you with support and instil within you a sense of confidence and belief in your own voice and in your capacity to create the best possible health outcome that is available for you and your loved ones.

Liz Crocker

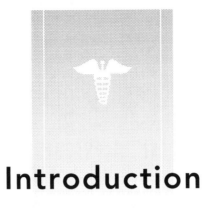

Introduction

THE PATIENT IS THE 'SUN' IN THE MEDICAL UNIVERSE

Your voice is important. If you only take one message from this Handbook, then please let it be this: you have a voice and you must learn how to use it effectively while you or someone you love is experiencing a health challenge if you are to achieve the best and safest outcome.

It was not always necessary for you to be as vocally active in your health care as it is today. Health care has changed. It is increasingly a system under strain. Decisions over limited health resources including questions of who can access health care, when, where, for how long, for what purpose and at whose cost are already complicated and will only become more so in the future.

We all need to learn how to speak up and participate in this new era of health care because the old ways of interacting will not always be as safe and effective as they used to be. This is despite the very best intentions and endeavours of the individual health care workers involved! The health system, which in many ways is like a machine, cannot always cater for the unique needs of the individual.

Health providers are increasingly seeking patients to become 'partners' in their health care. This sounds good – except that many patients and their families don't really understand what is now expected of them. It is still common for patients and families who, for obvious reasons, are in a state of vulnerability, to default to a passive role in their health care relationships. They can all too easily 'hand over' their personal power and decision-making capacity to the health provider and health system. This is especially the case for people who are older or who are not naturally assertive.

If patients and families do not know that the 'goal posts' have changed, then they are not going to be alert or prepared. They will continue to remain silent and defer to the health provider while trusting that 'all will work out in the end'. But it is this silence that often leads to unwanted consequences. These consequences are rarely any one person's fault – in most cases they are the result of small 'perfect storms' within a busy system that is trying to meet the needs of many with resources that are increasingly stretched.

The patient is the **only** constant factor in health care, and so patients need to learn to speak. Everything revolves around the patient. This is why they are the 'sun' in the medical universe. This is why the patient (or the patient's family, friend or representative) must find their voice. They need to be alert, engaged and vocal. They need to *know* that they have a vital role to play and be confident in *how* to play that role. This is the only way that patients can uphold their end of the bargain and be a true 'partner' in their health care.

This Handbook aims to give you practical ways to develop and use your voice. It is not about creating conflict or being the loudest voice in the room – it is about being the most effective. It is about having a strategy and using clear communication to create the best possible outcome that is available to you or your loved one in your specific circumstances.

This material was originally developed as a Training Course for people in Australia who were interested in patient advocacy. A patient advocate, as the name suggests, is someone who acts as a spokesperson or representative for patients and their families. The information in this Handbook has been modified from the original Course materials so it can be applied straight away. No prior learning is required!

Although this material is based on the Australian health care system, most of the information is generic and can therefore be applied in other jurisdictions as well. However, where any legal or specific terms are covered, please note that this will relate **only** to the Australian context and was accurate at the time the material was originally published. It is therefore essential to make your own enquiries before relying on this material in case anything has changed in this very dynamic field.

We have also included a number of links to external resources throughout this Handbook. All links were current at the time of publication, however links can easily change. For this reason we have also included some suggested 'search terms' which you can use in your internet browser to find a similar resource.

Finally, we know that you are probably reading this Handbook at a time when you are in a state of stress and anxiety. In Chapter 1 we have provided a summary of **what to do in the event of an emergency**. We have also kept the rest of the Handbook as simple and easy to apply as possible – including giving you practical Exercises to help you to build confidence and skill.

Above all, please remember that simply by speaking up, being alert and being involved you will already be making a real difference for yourself or someone you love as you move through the health system.

CHAPTER

1

IN THE EVENT OF AN EMERGENCY...

If you are dealing with an emergency you will not have the time or the mental space to read and absorb the material in this Handbook. **Below is a quick guide which we hope will assist you with whatever you are facing**. When the immediate crisis has passed, please come back and read the rest of this Handbook.

WHAT TO DO RIGHT NOW:

- Handle the practical elements of what is happening right now. Create safety.
- Stay calm and clear headed. Ignore your emotions. You need to focus.
- Follow the advice of health professionals. Call an ambulance if required.
- Handle each situation one step at a time.
- Gather key medical information (medications, allergies, blood type, insurances, relevant legal documents, etc).
- Stop momentum from taking hold. It is the enemy of good decision-making.
- Take notes of all key events, actions and advice (on paper or on your phone).
- Understand the financial consequences of each decision as much as possible.
- Pack a bag. Bring your phone charger but leave precious items and jewellery at home.
- Make sure your house is secured and that it is safe (oven, heaters, electric blankets etc are all turned off).
- Look after yourself where you can and accept help when it is offered.

HANDLE THE IMMEDIATE SITUATION

Stay calm, ignore your feelings and FOCUS. Right now – what needs to be done?

Follow the advice of health professionals. Does an ambulance need to be called? If so then call one – and make sure you give your location and details of what is happening to the operator as clearly as you can. Does a next of kin or friend of the person need to be informed? Then call them. Are you alone and in trouble? Then get yourself to a basic level of safety as best you can. Focus 100% on stabilising what is happening right now and creating safety. Handle one thing at a time.

Locate all relevant medical information for yourself or the person involved (such as current medications, blood type information, allergy information, health insurance details, legal documents (if any) concerning medical treatment etc). It is always good to have this information stored somewhere that is easy to access in the event of an emergency. If you do not have it or cannot find it then call a relative of the person and see if they know anything that could help you. Do the best you can.

Take notes. Write down what has happened and when. Write down the advice you have been given. Write down what the medical response has been. Keep track of medications, dosages and time frames. It is essential to keep track of everything in case it is needed later on.

If you or someone you love has just received bad medical news, then the same approach applies. You need to stabilise the current situation i.e. find somewhere to sit and absorb the initial shock. Do not drive, walk too far or engage with too many people until you are ready. Do not try and process what you have been told. Focus on achieving stability so you can get home or to your destination. Be very practical, ignore your feelings as much as you can for the time being and just handle the basics.

HANDLE YOURSELF

Continue to stay calm. You are probably in shock – but do not allow your emotions to take over. Be as steady as you can. Strange things may happen (you may put your car keys in the fridge!) Know that you are just in shock and it is okay. You must stay calm.

If you have the luxury of time (whether that be minutes, hours or days) then force yourself to stop and try to transition through the shock as best you can with the time you have available. Make a cup of tea or coffee (anything nurturing) and drink it. **Slow down**. Do not pretend to be able to work or perform normal tasks. Allow your psyche and body the chance to process what has happened and to adjust.

It is important to be as self-aware as you can be, without engaging too much in the emotional sphere. You have to remain clear in your mind and the emotional state can overwhelm you, so focus on stability, practicals and what is happening right now.

If there is someone steady who you can call and talk to, then call them and if they are close by ask them to come over. This may not be your best friend – you want the *right* friend. Someone who enjoys a drama is not the right person!

If you are going to a hospital pack a bag (both for yourself and for the patient if you are not the patient). Make sure you pack clothes, personal items, your phone charger and a book or something to help you to pass the time (there is a lot of time spent waiting in hospitals). Leave all jewellery/precious personal items safely at home. Turn off the oven, heaters, electric blankets etc so your home is safe. Remember to lock external doors and windows.

If you have a child or a pet that needs to be looked after while you go to the hospital, then arrange for someone you trust to help you. Arrange (or ask them to arrange) a trusted back-up support person if that is needed so you don't have to think about anything other than the health crisis. Do not believe you can do it all yourself. You need to bring in the best external support you can – as quickly as possible.

STOP THE MOMENTUM!

Momentum is the enemy of good decision making. It is astonishing how quickly momentum takes hold – especially in emergency situations and especially in the health sector. Momentum is the single most dangerous element you need to manage, because it can take hold like a runaway train. Your primary job is always to STOP THE MOMENTUM so that good decisions can be made at each stage of the process.

If you are facing a life-threatening situation, then you need to allow those who have expert knowledge to guide and advise you. Try to ignore your own feelings as much as you can (there is plenty of time for that later) and work to get the best outcome for the patient that is possible. Urgent decisions may need to be made, so you must keep yourself steady and your mind clear and focused.

If it isn't a life-threatening situation then there is TIME. You may not need to make a decision in this moment, so be polite but firm. **Take time**. This could be minutes, hours or days – but unless the situation demands urgency, you should work to create space and time. If you have just been given a diagnosis and you are being asked to book into surgery immediately – you can still take some time. Take as much time as you can to break the momentum, to allow the initial shock to pass and for clear thinking to return. If you cannot do this for yourself then bring in someone you trust to help you who can be more objective.

GAIN MORE INFORMATION

Health providers are required to obtain consent to perform medical treatment on a patient, and that consent must be given either by the patient or by the next appropriate person (which depends on the patient's situation). So, if you or the patient are not ready to make a decision – do not make one. Do not give consent to treatment until you are ready. This means you need to ask more questions, perhaps gain a second opinion, and give yourself time to reflect and think. Do not allow yourself to feel rushed into consenting to treatment.

If the decision you are facing has irreversible consequences then this is even more important. It is your body – you must know and understand what is happening and the choices available to you. All of the choices. You need to feel as comfortable as you can with the course of action that is being presented. Do not agree to treatment until you are ready. If your health team believes a delay will cause bad outcomes, then this is part of what you are considering. But you are still the 'boss' of your body, so you need to factor in all the options before making a decision.

Once again, time is the most important element to manage here. You need to find out how much time you can really take (not what suits other people) and then use that time well. If it is minutes, then take minutes. Force yourself to calm down and think. If you have hours, then take hours. If you have days, then take days. Take as much time as you can and need – because afterwards you will go over and over this in your mind, so you want to feel comfortable that every choice was the best choice for you.

THINK ABOUT MONEY

We know this may seem inappropriate, but money is an important factor in health care. Make sure you know what the financial consequences of different choices will be, and that you can manage it. Ask questions. What is the difference (including financial difference) between being a 'public' health patient or a 'private' health patient? What out-of-pocket costs are there likely to be? What options do you have?

You also need to manage your own financial and work sphere. If you are employed, you need to talk with your employer and arrange for leave. Keep them informed so they can help you to manage your work responsibilities. If you run your own business, it can be very challenging if you are a sole operator. Manage as best you can, and if you need someone to make calls to customers or clients for you then allow this to happen. Try and remember when the mortgage or car payments are due so you meet your obligations. It can be difficult, but this also creates stability. This is an area where someone else can really help you.

MAKE A DECISION

When you are free of momentum and as clear headed as possible, then make a decision. After weighing it all up and understanding all the choices before you, pick the best choice for you. Sometimes you can talk and reach agreement with other people, and sometimes you need to act alone and against the wishes of others. Either way, make sure your decision is your own and that you are comfortable with it.

This is not the time to seek approval. Whether the health provider agrees with you or not doesn't matter. It is your body, your choice. Whether your family or friends agree doesn't matter either. You need to make the choice you believe is right for you or for the person concerned if you are not the patient. This is not the time to worry about being liked or being harmonious. You need to make the right decision for the longer term.

GO THE DISTANCE

Some health journeys are a sprint, others are a marathon. Try and identify which one this will be, as this will help you to manage yourself and to build resilience.

You may have one difficult decision to make, or ten difficult decisions to make. If you think it's only one decision but it turns out to be ten, then by decision 'five' you will be tiring and by decision 'ten' you will have lost all clarity and focus. You need to build the internal capacity to make good decisions at decision 'one' *and* decision 'ten' – because every decision is important.

You also need to look after yourself (if you are not the patient) so you have the stamina to keep going. This means sleeping when you can, eating the best food you can, taking gentle walks to get fresh air and so on. Delegate as much of everyday life as possible. Say yes when people offer to help you – whether it's with the washing, paying bills, putting out the garbage, informing other people – you need to delegate and accept help wherever it is available to you. Do not try and handle it all alone.

GAIN SUPPORT

When it is all over, or at least when the situation has stabilised, then it is time for you to process your emotions and how you feel about what has happened. If you do not do this important step then it will most likely cause issues for you in some other part of your life, so make it a priority. To have handled what has happened you have had to ignore this emotional part of yourself – but now it needs expression and attention.

Find someone you can talk to. You need to process what has occurred, what it means to you and how you are handling it. This could be with family or friends, but if you have been through something serious and shocking then you are better to engage a professional. You might need one session or several, but you are giving yourself the best chance to move forward if you make this step important.

If you were the patient, then this is also an important step for you. Just because you are recovering physically does not mean you are recovering emotionally or psychologically. We are extremely complex beings who feel and process experiences on many levels. We urge you to make the mental and emotional part of you as important as the physical part of you. Be patient. Recovery takes time.

CHAPTER

2

YOU ARE NOW A PATIENT ADVOCATE!

If you are helping someone who is receiving medical treatment to navigate their way forward through the health system, then you are a patient advocate. This Handbook will help you to learn what to do, what not to do, and how to act in order to achieve the best outcome for the person who is the patient.

WHAT IS A PATIENT ADVOCATE?

An advocate is someone who speaks on behalf of, or promotes the interests of, another person. It is a word taken from the legal system.

There is no standard definition of a patient advocate. Terms such as patient advocate, health advocate, patient representative, patient navigator and patient facilitator are often used interchangeably. We define a patient advocate as follows:

> A patient advocate is someone who speaks for, acts on behalf of, or otherwise assists a person seeking access to, or receiving, health services – with the objective of helping that person to achieve the best health outcome that is available to them.

Patient advocacy as an *activity* has been around for centuries as people have always helped those they love in times of difficulty. However, patient advocacy as a *discipline* is believed to have emerged from the patients' rights movement in the United States in the early 1970s.[1]

EXAMPLES OF PATIENT ADVOCATES

Private Patient Advocates

A private or professional patient advocate is someone who is paid for their services directly by the patient or by someone on the patient's behalf, such as by a relative, friend or carer.

A private patient advocate should be completely focused on the needs of their client and should not have any conflict of interest or loyalty (through employment, commission or similar relationship) to any other organisation, business or employer.

Private patient advocacy businesses now exist in several countries including the United Kingdom, Ireland, Thailand, Vietnam, Spain and Australia – however the industry remains most established in the United States.

Patient Liaison Officers and Patient Representatives

Patient Liaison Officers (also called Patient Representatives) are often employed by a health service provider (such as a hospital, clinic or similar health service) to give assistance to patients while they are receiving services from that provider.

Patient Liaison Officers are very useful as the first point of call for patients and families and can provide significant assistance. It is however important to know that they are usually not independent from the health system. They are also often only available during certain hours.

Nurses

Nurses are extremely powerful and effective patient advocates. It is a key part of a nurse's role to express the concerns of a patient to other medical staff and to assist the patient and their family to understand what is said to them so they can make informed choices about their health care and treatment.

However, a nurse can only assist a patient while that patient is under their care. Once the patient is moved to a different ward, is discharged or is otherwise relocated, the nurse rarely has any further role with that patient. As employees of a health provider, nurses can also have an inherent conflict of interest between the patient and their employer. Finally, it is well understood that there are extremely high workload demands on nursing staff, especially in hospitals, which can limit the level of personal focus that is available for a particular patient.

Despite these complexities you should always aim to work as closely as possible with nurses as they are a tremendous source of support both for you and for the patient.

Consumer Health Organisations

Consumer health organisations are very effective and respected health advocates. These organisations usually focus on a specific health issue, illness/disease type or population sector (such as epilepsy, cancer, diabetes, HIV/AIDs, dementia, etc).

Consumer health organisations can provide enormous assistance by helping patients and families locate experienced health providers and support groups, and almost always this support is available free of charge. They are, however, generally less inclined to provide direct or in-person advocacy services.

Family, Friends and Carers

Family, friends and carers of patients are often the most effective patient advocates. They know the patient and are in the best position to observe and draw the attention of the health team to issues and changes in the patient. The patient is also usually more comfortable telling those close to them how they really feel and what is of concern to them.

Family, friends and carers also generally have no other loyalty or consideration beyond the patient.

WHAT DOES A PATIENT ADVOCATE DO?

Patient advocacy is usually a short-term activity. The assistance is immediate and of finite duration – if your mother is admitted into hospital, then your work as a 'patient advocate' for her begins the moment she is admitted and may finish once she returns home and is in recovery.

People generally know when they are vulnerable and need help. This vulnerability can stem from the person's health condition as well as from personal factors such as their age, gender, language, religion, cultural factors, sexuality or even from their personality type (for example if they are shy and non-assertive).

A patient advocate will provide the help and protection that the person is seeking through their ability to **negotiate**, **mediate** and, where necessary, **intercede** on behalf of that person in order to improve the health outcome that is achievable for them.

> This is what a patient advocate actually does: **negotiate**, **mediate** and **intercede**.

Each of these actions requires specific skills and techniques which we will explore in detail later in this Handbook. However, by way of introduction:

- **Negotiate** – this is the ability to find a way to take a practical action that will move the case forward. It can be making calls or researching options that are available, as well as speaking on behalf of a patient to facilitate a future collaboration between different health providers, particularly at different stages of the health care process.

- **Mediate** – this is when there are interpersonal and/or resource-based conflicts or challenges, for example, when there are a number of parties entrenched in a particular position and it appears that no solution can be found. In these situations, the advocate will work to build a new 'common ground' between the parties to create a forward movement for the patient.

- **Intercede** – sometimes it is necessary to directly intercede for a patient. This involves creating a 'wedge' in the flow of health care that the patient is receiving. The advocate is effectively 'stopping the momentum' on behalf of the patient. In some cases there is no immediate risk of impact to the patient, but some intervention on their behalf is required. In other cases a patient may be about to receive medical treatment (for example surgery), but may want the process stopped or slowed down.

WHAT SHOULD A PATIENT ADVOCATE NOT DO?

If someone is acting as a private (i.e. paid) patient advocate, then they should never do the following:

- Make a medical treatment decision for, or on behalf of, a patient;
- Tell the patient what decision they should make in relation to medical treatment;
- Assume the role of being the substitute decision-maker for the patient;
- Make or offer any kind of medical diagnosis;
- Treat or provide medical care to a patient;
- Provide legal advice of any kind to a patient or other person; or
- Assume the role of counsellor or social worker for the patient.

If you are helping a family member or friend, then this is obviously not the case. You will naturally provide personal support to someone you love and care about. You may also be their substitute decision-maker in the decision-making hierarchy (see later in this Handbook), or you might be their medical representative.

In each situation it is important to always make sure that you *know* which 'hat' you are wearing: are you speaking and acting as a 'daughter', or as a 'patient advocate'?

LEGAL REGULATION OF PATIENT ADVOCACY

Currently anyone with legal capacity over 18 years of age can be a patient advocate in Australia. There are some further legal requirements if you are seeking to work as a private (professional) patient advocate with certain groups, such as with children.

At the time of writing, there is no common regulation, licensing, certification or other supervision of private patient advocates. However, although the industry appears quite fragmented, there is some movement especially in the United States to create a formal certification system for patient advocates.

In the absence of this regulation, universities, medical schools, professional organisations and private institutes are taking up the challenge to educate and provide a system of quality assurance for the benefit of patients and families.

KEY LEARNINGS FROM CHAPTER 2

- You are a patient advocate if you are helping someone who is receiving health care – regardless of whether you are being paid or not!
- The three key roles of a patient advocate are to negotiate, mediate and/or to intercede on behalf of a patient.
- Patient advocacy is an emerging industry that is developing around the world.
- If you are wishing to pursue patient advocacy as a profession there may be additional legal, regulatory and related requirements that apply in your country.

PRACTICE EXERCISE – CHAPTER 2

Please read the following three Case Studies:

Mary

Mary, aged 48, was the victim of a serious incapacitation and had been admitted to a leading metropolitan hospital for rehabilitation. Hers was a difficult case with little hope that she would recover any significant prior mobility. She had previously lived with her husband on a farm in country Victoria. Her husband was unable to travel, and they were becoming increasingly distressed, both due to the separation and the cost for her husband to live in temporary accommodation in Melbourne.

The family had tried to talk to the hospital but were (in their view) not being taken seriously. As their stress level increased, so did the level of conflict with hospital staff over what was best for Mary. A private patient advocate was engaged by Mary's daughter and, with Mary's permission, a meeting was scheduled between the treating doctors, relevant nursing staff and the family to discuss all potential options for Mary's care and treatment.

After a full exchange of concerns and views, the hospital agreed to actively facilitate Mary's transfer to a regional hospital closer to her home, on the condition that appropriate rehabilitation care could be provided by the regional hospital. This was arranged. Mary was then transferred, and her health improved.

Andrew

Andrew was 40 years of age and had undergone 14 surgical operations on his right knee following an earlier sporting injury. He was scheduled to have a further operation, however he was in chronic pain and seriously considering the amputation of his leg above the knee. On the advice of a friend, he contacted a private patient advocate.

The advocate spent considerable time working through Andrew's case history to determine what (if any) dispute existed between different medical practitioners and providers to account for his continued pain. The advocate then arranged for an independent surgeon to review the case and provide advice. On the advice of the new surgeon, Andrew cancelled his upcoming surgery and engaged a physiotherapist to collaborate with the surgeon to oversee a radically different treatment strategy. Under the coordinated care of these practitioners, the movement in Andrew's knee began to improve and his pain level began to recede.

Daniel

Daniel suffered from a lung disease which necessitated regular but unplanned trips to the emergency department of a local hospital, generally at night. He contacted a private patient advocate for help because he found that his condition often worsened while he sat in the emergency waiting room.

His advocate worked with the hospital and discovered that a new 'Health Alert' system had been introduced which could be utilised to assist Daniel on admission. The advocate worked with Daniel's treating specialist and the relevant personnel at the hospital to create a new in-take procedure that would enable Daniel to immediately receive treatment whenever he presented at emergency.

After a recent admission, Daniel contacted his advocate to say that the new procedure had worked extremely well as he had been able to get the care he needed faster (and be discharged sooner) and with less intensive medical intervention than had previously been the case.

Please answer the following two questions:

1. Which was the dominant action taken by the private patient advocate in each of these three Cases? Was it: a) to **negotiate**, b) to **mediate** or c) to **intercede**?

Some 'example answers' for this question are included at the end of this Handbook.

2. Which of these three actions - **negotiate, mediate** or **intercede** - do you feel is most natural for you? And which do you feel is the most challenging?

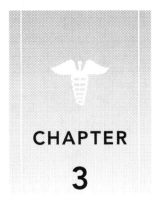

CHAPTER

3

KNOW YOUR RIGHTS
(PART 1 – HEALTH POLICY)

It is always easier to assert yourself if you know that you are 'in the right'. You might know the health system. You might know the law. You might follow a particular moral or ethical philosophy or have some other platform of knowledge that gives you certainty. If you own a shop and know that 'stealing is wrong', then you will feel empowered to call the police if you observe a shoplifter. Or if the shoplifter knows that they have the right to speak with a lawyer when they are arrested, then they will feel confident waiting for their lawyer to arrive before answering any questions.

It is the same with health care. If you are confident in your position, then it is easier to speak up for what you want and to express your concerns. But if you are unsure, then you may be more inclined to hesitate, remain quiet and be more compliant.

In this Chapter we will start to build the platform for your own patient advocacy. This means we will help you to understand some of the rights patients have so you know when and how to think, speak and act when navigating the health system. We will introduce you to some important aspects of health **policy** that is relevant to patient care, and in the next Chapter we will explore some of the **law** relating to this area.

Please note that although many of the broad principles will be relevant to health care in other countries, the information contained in this Chapter and in the next Chapter is very specific to Australia. This Handbook should also not be taken in any way as providing specific legal advice as it is very general in nature. Great care should therefore be taken in relying upon this information without gaining further advice specific to your unique situation and jurisdiction.

THE DIFFERENCE BETWEEN LAW AND POLICY

The delivery of health care services in Australia (and in many other countries) is governed by *both* law and policy. The law, although powerful and certain, is by its nature very slow, limited and inflexible. This is because, in Australia, it depends either on a parliament passing legislation, or on a court or tribunal to decide a case with factual circumstances specific enough to address a particular issue and with sufficient authority to influence future behaviour.

By contrast, policy is highly flexible and can be adjusted relatively easily to respond to changing social priorities, attitudes and circumstances. It is much more dynamic, but it is also much less certain. Due in part to this inherent flexibility, the majority of health care in Australia is managed through policy and *not* through the law.

> Understanding the difference between law and policy is essential if you are to be an effective patient advocate because this influences the **power balance** that exists between you and the health system – and therefore the options and solutions that will be available to you.

If a patient's legal right is infringed, then they are usually in a strong position with clear options available to them. This is because the legal system takes legal rights very seriously and has mechanisms in place to address any breaches. It is also an important principle of the law that legal rights should be as clear and certain as possible, so these areas tend to be more 'black and white'. So, when you know the law is on your side, you can be more confident and assured in your communication, expectations and decisions.

Most areas of health care are, however, governed by policy. Policy is very discretionary which means it is open to the decision-maker to decide 'yes or no' based on the circumstances before them. Provided their exercise of discretion is reasonable, then other than complain about it afterwards there is often little that can be done because the decision-maker has simply prioritised one area of policy over another. This uncertainty is a key disadvantage that flows from the flexibility of policy. It is much more of a 'grey zone', and so it is likely you will feel less confident and less assured when dealing with matters governed by health policy.

This is why it is essential to always know the platform for your advocacy: are you standing on solid rock or on a flimsy bridge? Do you have an actual right that you can assert? Or do you need to convince someone in authority to see an issue from your point of view? These positions are very different! The way you manage yourself and the patient you are helping will depend upon the answer. Finally, it is not always easy to know if a situation is governed by policy or by law because, as will be shown below, many health policies use legal language!

In the rest of this Chapter we will therefore explore some key aspects of Australian health policy from the perspective of patient advocacy. This material may appear dry – but understanding the *language and priorities* of health providers and what *they* consider to be important will greatly assist you in your own advocacy.

IS THERE A 'RIGHT' TO HEALTH?

Health as an *objective* is governed entirely by policy in Australia. There are currently no legally enforceable rights to access health care in any legislation at any level of government in Australia.[2] A 'legally enforceable' right is a right that enables a person who believes that their right has been infringed to apply to a court or to a tribunal for assistance. This might be through, for example, getting an order requiring a provider to act in a particular way, to do a certain thing, or to have compensation paid.

Australia is one of the few modern democracies in the world that does not have any express protection for human rights in its Constitution. It is important to be aware of this because Australia is a highly developed country and has a very individualistic culture. Patients and families can therefore easily assume that legal rights in this area exist and are 'owed' to them, when this is not actually the case!

Through its agreement to international human rights law instruments, Australia must however *observe* human rights, some of which relate to health. In particular, the *International Covenant on Economic, Social and Cultural Rights* (ICESCR), to which Australia is a party, recognises *"the right of everyone to the enjoyment of the highest attainable standard of physical and mental health."*[3]

The United Nations' Committee on Economic, Social and Cultural Rights has stated that the right to health is not to be understood as a right to be healthy, and it does not require governments to establish health care systems beyond their means.[4] The notion of *"the highest attainable standard of physical and mental health"* takes into account a country's available resources, and so developed countries (such as Australia) are held to higher standards by the international community than developing countries.[5]

Although Australia is a party to the ICESCR, there is no legislation expressly enshrining the right to health in Australia.[6] It is considered to be more of an *aspirational* objective.

AUSTRALIAN CHARTER OF HEALTHCARE RIGHTS

The *Australian Charter of Healthcare Rights* (the Charter) applies to all health settings anywhere in Australia, including publicly and privately funded hospitals and general practice clinics.[7] Although the Charter uses the term 'rights' extensively, it is in fact a statement of health policy. The Charter allows patients, consumers, families, carers and providers to share an understanding of the rights of people receiving health care and is considered to be a very important document in the Australian health industry.

There are three Guiding Principles that underpin the Charter:

1. Everyone has the right to be able to access health care and this right is essential for the Charter to be meaningful.
2. The Australian Government commits to international agreements about human rights which recognise everyone's right to have the highest possible standard of physical and mental health.
3. Australia is a society made up of people with different cultures and ways of life, and the Charter acknowledges and respects these differences.[8]

The Charter contains seven 'Charter Rights', which are as follows:

- Access: I have a right to health care.
- Safety: I have a right to receive safe and high quality care.
- Respect: I have a right to be shown respect, dignity and consideration.
- Communication: I have a right to be informed about services, treatment, options and costs in a clear and open way.
- Participation: I have a right to be included in decisions and choices about care.
- Privacy: I have a right to privacy and confidentiality of my personal information.
- Comment: I have a right to comment on my care and have my concerns addressed.[9]

The Charter is important because the 'rights' and concepts contained within it reflect the values and priorities contained in a significant volume of health care policy. It is therefore very useful to become familiar with the language and concepts so you can communicate effectively within the health system.

Although this information is specific to Australia, it is likely that similar language will be used in health policies in other countries. For this reason, each of the seven 'Charter Rights' are explained in further detail below:[10]

Access

Access is the right to receive health care. According to the Charter, there is a fundamental right to adequate and timely health care, regardless of gender, marital status, disability, culture, religious beliefs, sexual orientation, age or geographic location. However, it is acknowledged that not all services are available in all areas.

Access – and how health services are financed – are closely tied. The right of access is facilitated in Australia primarily through Medicare which helps to provide patients with free or subsidised access to medical treatment, including through public hospitals. When the required treatment resources are not available locally, the patient will be transferred or referred to a service able to deliver appropriate care. Non-emergency care may require a patient to wait for treatment, depending on the urgency and the availability of the care required.

Under the Charter, health providers should discuss any issues concerning access with the patient to encourage informed choice, but must also act to ensure the efficient use of services and implement timely discharge processes to enable access by others. Health providers need to ensure that adequate facilities, equipment and supplies are available so that staff can provide services in a timely and appropriate fashion, ensure the efficient management of beds and facilities to optimise access, provide an opportunity for patients to choose whether to be treated as a 'public' or 'private' patient and to explain that choice, provide support (where appropriate) for people who need to travel to receive public health care services, and ensure transparency and accountability in all decisions about access.

Safety

Patients have the right to safe and high-quality care, and patients and health care providers are entitled to a safe, secure and supportive health care environment. In some areas this means patients will receive health care on the basis of their assessed need regardless of their financial situation and that those patients who are sickest will be treated first. In other areas this means the right to be safe from abuse or the risk of abuse, the right for patients to have their legal and human rights respected and upheld, and for services provided to patients to comply with legal, professional, ethical and other relevant standards.

The right to safe and high-quality health care relies in part on clear communication. Patients need to express any safety concerns they might have, such as by informing treating medical staff if they think something has been missed in their care or if an error has occurred. Patients have a right to an accredited interpreter when using a public health care service to improve communication, which also contributes to patient safety.

Health providers need to provide health services with professional skill, care and competence, which means provide services that are based on evidence of safety and effectiveness and work to provide continuity of care for patients. Health providers need to employ appropriately qualified staff and managers, ensure that facilities and procedures meet industry standards, provide staff with necessary resources and put systems in place that promote patient safety. All health providers should work to continually improve their safety and quality of care.

Respect

All participants in the health care system are entitled to be treated with respect and not be discriminated against in any way, including by race, age, gender, gender identity, sexual orientation, carer status, disability, marital status or religious belief. Patients have a right to receive care in a manner that is respectful of their culture, beliefs and values. This may include beliefs and practices around birth, illness and death, the gender of the person treating them and their dietary requirements while in hospital.

As far as possible, health providers should offer care and treatment in surroundings that allow personal privacy. The right is also described to mean patients have a right to receive visitors and to be given privacy. There is also the ability for people with guide dogs to visit patients as well as other visits involving pets as approved by the health provider.

Patients need to respect the well-being and rights of other patients, consumers and staff. They should let staff know if there have been changes to their condition or any new symptoms and if they have been unable to follow their health plans. Staff and health service managers are also entitled to be treated politely and with consideration of their workload. This right is also seen to be applied through patients, staff and visitors being asked to respect visiting hours, infection control measures, smoke-free zones and limitations around the use of mobile phones around medical equipment.

Health providers need to demonstrate professional conduct that is based on ethical standards and treat patients with dignity and consideration. This includes providing care in a manner that is respectful of a person's culture and beliefs and is free from discrimination, as well as interacting with clinical colleagues, paramedical and service staff and managers in a respectful manner. Health providers need to develop and maintain a co-operative and mutually respectful environment to support interactions between patients and staff, as well as support staff to abide by agreed and published ethical standards, practices and professional codes of conduct.

Communication

Patients have a right to be fully informed about all aspects of their health care including what options are available, expected outcomes, information about side effects, where the services would be provided and the costs of the service – and for all of this information to be communicated in a clear and comprehensible way. In some jurisdictions the Charter right to communication expressly states that if a patient has concerns about their treatment options, they can obtain a second medical opinion. Patients in a hospital or other large health care service where they may be treated by a number of people have a right to be kept informed about who is responsible for their care, and how to best contact them.

In order to obtain the best possible health outcome, the exchange of information between patients and staff must be full and open. Patients should have the opportunity to ask questions if more information about any aspect of care is needed. Patients should be as open and honest with staff as possible, including giving details of their medical history and medication they may be taking (including complementary therapies), as well as details of their social circumstances and emotional well-being. This assists the health provider to offer the patient the most appropriate treatment. Patients are also encouraged to tell their health care provider the name and contact details of the person who can provide consent if the patient is not able to do so.

Health providers need to provide patients and consumers with open, complete and timely communication throughout the period of care, including when plans change or if something goes wrong. They need to ensure the appropriate transfer of information when care is handed over to another health provider. Health providers also need to provide patients with advice on how and where to ask questions and obtain information about diagnosis and treatment from their health care team, make all reasonable efforts to afford access to services such as interpreters and patient support groups and provide information about the facility's waiting times and costs of services. Finally, they should ensure that there is a continuity of service providers and have systems in place to support open disclosure when things go wrong.

Participation

To obtain good health outcomes, it is important for patients and consumers to participate in decisions and choices about their care and health needs. This provides the basis for consent and informed decision making. Patients need to participate as fully as they can in the decisions about their care and treatment. This means the patient's family can be actively involved, the patient can seek a second opinion if they have any uncertainty, they can give or withhold permission for treatment and can involve their family, carers or another nominated support person to support their decision making. Many of these aspects of health care are addressed in further detail in the next Chapter of this Handbook.

The right to participation has been described to mean that patients have a right to be fully involved in decisions and choices about health services. They have a right to support and advocacy, and a right to seek advice or information from other sources. Patients have a right to give, withhold or withdraw their consent at any time. Patients have the right, where circumstances permit, to have a relative or support person with them at all times, they have the right to decline having a student present while their care is being provided, the right to withhold consent to medical treatment, the right to refuse to be part of health and medical research and the right to talk to their general practitioner and seek a second medical opinion. In Victoria these rights are expressed as follows:

- You have a right to take an active role in your health care and to be included in decisions and choices about your care;
- You have a right to participate as fully as you wish in decisions about your care and treatment. Your health care provider should give you all the information you need to make informed decisions, the opportunity to ask questions, and time to talk to your carers, family and friends before making decisions;
- You have a right to have your family, other carers or chosen support person involved in your care. With your consent, they can also receive information and be involved in making decisions about your care with you;
- You have a right to refuse treatment. However, there are circumstances in which you may be regarded as unable to give informed consent or to refuse treatment;

- You have a right to appoint someone to make medical decisions for you in the event that you lose the capacity to do so; and
- If you are a hospital patient, you have a right to be involved in the decision about how and when you leave hospital. Before you leave, the hospital should discuss what health care services you may need after you leave hospital and refer you to them. You have a right to participate in decisions about your ongoing care. Your GP should also be involved. You may discharge yourself against your doctor's advice, but you may be asked to sign a form accepting responsibility for this.

Health providers need to encourage patients to make fully informed decisions by discussing treatment options available including expected outcomes, success rates and incidence of side effects. They need to inform patients of their right to refuse treatment or withdraw consent at any time. They must ensure patients are especially aware of any care or treatment offered to them that is experimental or part of teaching or research. Health providers need to develop and maintain policies that encourage and appropriately support patients and their families to be involved in decision-making and facilitate the involvement of patients in decisions regarding health service policies and planning.

Privacy

Everyone participating in the health care system needs to respect the privacy of other people in the health system, and everyone involved in the patient's treatment and care has a professional and legal duty to keep information about the patient confidential.

Patients have a right to expect that their personal health information will be collected, used, disclosed and stored in accordance with the relevant laws about privacy, and that this information will remain confidential unless the law allows disclosure or the individual directs otherwise. They also have the right to say what happens to their information. If they decide not to share some of their information this is their right – but it may affect their health provider's ability to provide the patient with the best possible care. A patient also has a right to access their health care record. If a patient is given only part of their record they have the right to apply for their complete record. Patients can nominate person/s with whom their health information can be shared.

Health providers need to ensure that patients' health information is only shared with other appropriate health care providers, recognise that patients have a right to access their records, be prepared to discuss the contents of their records with them and be sensitive to the privacy needs of patients. Health providers need to ensure that procedures are in place so that information about patients is treated in confidence. Facilities must be available to secure health records, provide systems to support patients to access their personal health information where permitted under relevant legislation and ensure procedures are in place to assist staff to understand the privacy rights of others, and what information they can disclose to whom.

Comment

According to the Charter, all participants in the health care system benefit from processes that encourage feedback about the services received by patients and encourage any concerns to be resolved in an open, fair and timely manner. If patients wish to provide feedback, they should first try to use the procedures and systems in the relevant organisation.

Patients have the right to seek to have their concerns resolved by independent arbitrators such as health care complaints commissions or through the legal system. Patients also have a right to a representative of their choice to support and advocate for them when making a complaint. Health care services should make information about their feedback processes easy to find. In a hospital, if a patient is unsatisfied with how their doctor or treatment team is responding to their concerns, they have a right to speak to the hospital's patient representative.

Health providers need to acknowledge and take seriously all comments and feedback made by patients. This requires them to establish feedback channels that are available at all times, facilitate the efficient and equitable resolution of complaints and establish 'reflective practices' to consider issues arising from comment to determine possible improvements. Health providers need to have a complaints handling system in place that operates according to best practice ensures that patients have access to information about the comment process without having to ask for it. It should also have a quality improvement system in place that considers the issues emerging from complaints and ensures processes exist for health care staff to also make complaints about their workplace and have their concerns acted on.

ENFORCING HEALTH POLICY –
WHAT ARE YOUR OPTIONS?

The 'rights' contained in the Charter are, in general, statements of policies and practices that *should* occur. Similar to the international human rights instruments, the Charter is aspirational in nature and so is not easy to directly enforce.

However – just because a right is contained in a policy and is not a 'legal' right does not mean you are without any options.

The options are just not as clear or as strong as when the law is infringed.

First, policies should be followed, and they should also be applied fairly and consistently. This means you can lobby for a policy (such as a right contained in the Charter) to be applied to you or your loved one in the same way that it has been applied for others. If you can show that 'event X' happened for Mr Jones, then it is very difficult for the hospital to say that 'event X' should not happen for Mr Smith. Or if a policy says that dogs are allowed in certain designated areas, then there should be a compelling reason why your dog cannot be brought in to visit you in that same designated area. Policies should be followed wherever possible.

> Knowing that these health policies exist and that you are (in principle) entitled to the 'rights' contained within them is a very powerful and important foundation for your patient advocacy. This is why you need to read them and learn their 'language'.

Second, there are often competing policies. For example, the right to access health care services is balanced with the right of other patients to access those same health care services. The health provider is generally the decision-maker around how this delicate balance should be managed. You may, through your effective and informed negotiation skills, be able to 'tip the balance' in their mind in order to achieve a specific outcome for you or for your loved one.

Finally, if a Charter 'right' has been breached or not complied with, you can make a formal complaint. Although there is no guarantee that anything will change, there is a greater chance of a different outcome than if you simply remain quiet. Engaging the support of the Patient Representative in a hospital can also be very effective.

In each case, knowing that health policies exist and contain these 'rights' provides you with part of the platform for your advocacy. It helps you to discern if you should (or can) **negotiate**, **mediate** and/or **intercede** in order to achieve a specific outcome.

KEY LEARNINGS FROM CHAPTER 3

- There is a difference between legal rights and policy-based rights. Knowing the difference determines the platform for your advocacy and the options that may be available to you.
- Although policy-based rights are not as strong as legal rights, it is still possible to create very positive outcomes if you know that these policies exist and what they say.
- It is very important to learn some of the key words and concepts used in health policy, as this may increase the likelihood of your request being favourably considered.

PRACTICE EXERCISE – CHAPTER 3

Jessica is 70 years old and has been admitted as a patient in a public hospital.

Please invent any personal or health characteristics for Jessica that you wish, and then select <u>one</u> of the seven rights contained in the *Australian Charter of Healthcare Rights*. Think of some practical actions that demonstrate how the right you have selected could be represented in a meaningful way for Jessica.

This Exercise may help you to think creatively about how policy documents like this can be used to help someone in a way that is practical and meaningful for them.

Some suggested answers to this Exercise can be found at the end of this Handbook.

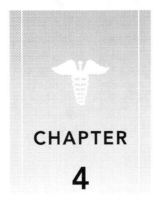

CHAPTER

4

KNOW YOUR RIGHTS
(PART 2 – LEGAL RIGHTS)

In addition to the policy-based rights introduced in Chapter 3, patients also have very specific legal rights in relation to receiving health services in Australia. This Chapter will introduce you to some of these rights to help you to build confidence in voicing your wishes and concerns while you or someone you love is receiving health services.

WHAT ARE LEGAL RIGHTS?

Legal rights are rights which are created either by legislation or by the common law. Legislation is passed by politicians in parliament. The common law is formed over a long period of time by judges in courts deciding what should happen in specific factual cases. These principles are then applied to similar factual cases that later arise, so over time the law becomes clear.

Due to historical factors, the common law in Australia is heavily influenced by decisions made in the United Kingdom. This is why there are often similarities in the law between countries which are (or were) part of the British Commonwealth (such as Australia, South Africa, Canada, New Zealand, India and so on).

In Chapter 3 we introduced you to the *Australian Charter of Healthcare Rights* (the Charter). As you will see below, although the Charter *itself* is not legally enforceable (because it has not been adopted or included in legislation), the Charter does incorporate several common law rights that *are* legally enforceable. This means that a breach of the Charter may be able to be enforced via the common law – *if* you are willing to take the matter to a court or a tribunal for assistance.

Most people understandably wish to avoid taking formal legal action, and we support this approach. Legal action should always be the last resort. In addition to being stressful and expensive, in most cases the harm to the person has already been done. It is much better to learn how to assert your legal rights *before or at the time the breach is occurring* so you can achieve the outcome you actually want. **Being 'right' afterwards is not as satisfactory as getting the right result when it matters.**

This is why understanding some of the key legal rights that apply to patients can help to make your advocacy much more effective.

CONSENT AND THE RIGHT TO REFUSE MEDICAL TREATMENT

One of the most important legal rights all patients have is the right to decide what happens to their own body. In legal terms this is called the law of consent and it includes the right to refuse medical treatment. We will deal with consent and refusal of treatment separately.

What is Consent?

The starting position in relation to consent to medical treatment is that **no medical treatment should be provided to any person without that person giving consent (that is, agreeing) to the provision of that treatment.**[11] To quote a highly regarded case from the United States which has since been endorsed in many other countries, including Australia:

> "Every human being of adult years and sound mind has a right to determine what shall be done with his own body; and a surgeon who performs an operation without his patient's consent, commits an assault, for which he is liable in damages."[12]

The main exception to this rule is in emergency situations where it may not be possible to obtain a patient's consent, but medical intervention is still considered to be necessary *and* reasonable.[13]

This legal right to be free from non-consensual medical treatment is considered an essential human right, and in some jurisdictions in Australia this right is also protected in legislation.[14]

Proper consent to medical treatment requires three main elements:

1. That the patient has the capacity to make treatment decisions;
2. That the consent they give is given freely and voluntarily; and
3. That the consent covers the act to be performed.[15]

Specific issues relating to the first requirement (including consent by people who are especially vulnerable, such as children, the elderly, people from non-English speaking backgrounds and people without capacity) are addressed later in this Chapter.

For people who are of adult years and of sound mind (which in the law means having 'capacity')[16], the second requirement relating to voluntariness is often seen as the most complex and controversial component of consent.

The third requirement, namely that the consent is specific and covers the act to be performed, is to protect patients from giving general or 'blanket consents'.[17] This means a health provider cannot assume that just because a patient agreed to one procedure that they will agree to the next procedure. It is a protection against momentum because each procedure must be independently consented to by the patient – one at a time (with limited exceptions for emergency situations).

The Meaning of 'Voluntary'

As stated above, each consent must be given by the patient freely and voluntarily. But what does this really mean?

The key to a truly voluntary decision is that the patient must not feel unduly influenced, pressured or manipulated into making a decision.[18] So, although the patient may be of sound mind, understand what is being said to them and even appear to agree that the treatment should proceed, the consent may still not actually be free or voluntary in the eyes of the law.

For example, a patient may feel that they have no choice but to consent to treatment in case questioning or refusing it means (in their mind) that other care won't be provided to them. They may fear that they could be labelled 'a difficult patient' and then be 'punished' in some way. This might be through not being taken to the toilet quickly enough or being left in the shower for too long. The deep vulnerability patients feel can make them believe they can't say 'no', even if they are not comfortable with the course of action that is proposed.

Alternatively, a patient may agree to treatment simply because they are trying to please their family and keep everyone happy. This is not 'free consent' either. It is up to families and friends as much as it is up to the health system to ensure that each patient decides what is right for them – as free of undue influence as possible.

Finally, the circumstances around the patient may impact on the voluntariness of the decision. If a patient is being asked to consent to treatment while they are being wheeled in a hospital bed to surgery, they are likely to feel a pressure to say 'yes'. Or if their doctor appears too busy to stop and discuss alternative treatments they may agree to go ahead just to keep everyone else happy. These are *practical* factors that impact on the voluntariness of consent. As expressed in a leading case from England, the key question is:

> "Does the patient really mean what he says or is he merely saying it for a quiet life, to satisfy someone else or because the advice and persuasion to which he has been subjected is such that he can no longer think and decide for himself? ..."[19]

The Information Required for Consent

For a consent to be considered free and voluntary patients need to be free of undue influence, be given the right information, and then have the time to consider and absorb that information – including the ability to seek further information and to ask questions if this is what they need to do.[20]

It is very easy to become overwhelmed and confused with medical information, and so the information given to a patient needs to be 'patient focused'.[21] This means it needs to be the information the patient requires, not the information the health system *thinks* a patient requires.[22] This information should cover basic matters such as how the treatment will be given, possible outcomes from the treatment, risks related to the treatment including possible side effects, alternative options available, financial considerations of the treatment and so on.[23] It can also include detail on the personal experience and success rate of the individual doctor so the patient can decide whether to seek out someone more experienced.[24]

Until a patient feels that they have the information *they* need to provide a 'free and voluntary' consent, they should not give consent to the medical treatment. However, if the situation is an emergency then the patient will need to balance the risk of action (without all the information they may wish) with the risk of delaying medical treatment.

Patients can seek advice from another medical practitioner (which is called getting a second opinion) to assist them in becoming sufficiently informed about their treatment decision. However, as shown in Chapter 3, policy concerns relating to access to health care may influence who should *pay* for this second opinion.

For example, if a patient in Australia would like a second opinion in the form of specialist advice, they may *request* a referral to the specialist from their doctor. Their doctor is not however *required* to provide a referral. This does not prevent the patient from seeing the specialist, but they will not be able to claim a benefit for the treatment under Medicare without the referral. This is how policies relating to accessing medical services impact on practical outcomes. The patient can still *access* the specialist, but they may have to *pay* for this privately and without a subsidy from the government.

Another example is if a patient is admitted in a public hospital and is seeking a second opinion. The hospital may not object to the patient getting this second opinion, but they may not agree to pay if the second doctor is from outside the hospital. If the patient cannot physically leave the hospital to consult with the specialist, then getting the specialist to come to the hospital could be very difficult. In these circumstances the patient may prefer to seek a second opinion from another doctor within the hospital who can more easily access the patient and their information. This is why having a basic understanding of your legal rights (and how these rights operate within a policy environment) is so important.

Consent Forms

Many health providers now ask patients to sign a consent form prior to medical treatment. It is not strictly necessary to sign a form as many 'consents' to treatment are given verbally or are even implied (such as when the patient holds out their arm for their blood pressure to be taken). [25] However, these forms are common for more serious procedures.

The decision to provide consent to treatment is one of the most important decisions a patient will make and should not be made lightly or under pressure. Signing the consent form is often the **practical action** that a patient will undertake to demonstrate or show the health provider that this consent has been given.

The consent form is therefore an important document and should not be signed until the patient is ready to give consent 'freely and voluntarily'.

> The requirement for consent to be provided in advance of medical treatment is one of the most powerful protections for patients in health systems around the world.

Right to Refuse Medical Treatment

The other aspect of the law of consent is the right to *refuse* medical treatment.

Patients have the right to refuse medical treatment **at any time**. As stated in one decision *"...a valid refusal may be based upon religious, social or moral grounds, or indeed on no apparent rational grounds; and is entitled to respect... regardless."*[26] This right to refuse medical treatment is also protected in legislation.[27]

A patient's decision to refuse medical treatment must not be dismissed simply because the doctor does not agree with (or does not understand) the patient's decision. It does not matter whether the reasons for refusal are *"...rational, irrational, unknown or even non-existent."*[28] Provided the patient has capacity (or has clearly stated their wishes in a valid advanced health directive which we will explore shortly), their refusal to treatment must be respected.

Patients may also change their mind at any time. A patient may decide not to proceed with medical treatment that they previously agreed to, and if they have refused medical treatment the patient can decide that they wish to receive that same treatment after all. This point is very important. Provided the patient has capacity, it is for the *patient* to decide what (if any) treatment they receive, and they have the right to change their mind about their treatment at any stage on their health journey.[29]

The right to refuse medical treatment becomes complicated when the consequence of the refusal is that the patient will die. It is however the patient's right to refuse treatment, and for this to result in death – provided the patient has capacity (or had capacity at the time of making a valid advanced health directive) and has been given all necessary and relevant information.[30] They should not be prevented from exercising their right to refuse treatment even if death is the outcome.

There is some legal complexity about what 'medical treatment' really means. It was traditionally the view that artificial nutrition and hydration constituted 'palliative care' and not 'medical treatment', which meant it was not possible for a patient to refuse this being provided. This is however now changing, so that palliative care can be refused which then allows a patient to die. [31] Each case depends entirely on the jurisdiction and the medical situation of the patient concerned.

Finally, there is a very important difference between euthanasia and the right to refuse medical treatment that results in death. To put it simply, the right to refuse medical treatment resulting in death is essentially an act of choice that allows the natural process of dying to proceed without intervention from the health system. It is the *prevention* of a positive action that extends life. By contrast, euthanasia involves a positive action or intervention that will bring around or accelerate death. These are treated very differently in the law.

ADVANCED HEALTH DIRECTIVES AND SUBSTITUTE DECISION-MAKERS

An advanced health directive is a document that outlines the medical care and treatment decisions a person wants made in the event that they lose capacity and cannot make their own medical treatment decisions at the necessary time. It is sometimes called a 'living will'.[32]

An advanced health directive may be used to request and to refuse medical treatment. Directives that request medical treatment are complicated because a doctor cannot be compelled to perform medical treatment that they consider to be futile.[33] The weight to be applied to a 'request' for treatment will therefore depend on the situation.

The key to a valid advanced health directive is that the person who makes the directive must have legal capacity and be free from undue influence at the time it is made.[34] The directive should also relate to the circumstances that occur.[35] It does not matter that the person subsequently loses capacity – if capacity existed when the directive was made, then it should be binding.

In addition to advanced health directives, a person may appoint a substitute decision-maker to make medical treatment decisions on their behalf in the event that they should lose capacity. Such persons are referred to as enduring attorneys, enduring guardians or medical agents under the various Acts of legislation that apply. It is always necessary to understand what is permitted in your specific jurisdiction.

In the event that a person has lost capacity, has not made an advanced health directive and has not appointed a substitute decision-maker, then there must still be a decision-maker in relation to medical care and treatment decisions. In these situations, a 'default decision-maker' will be appointed under the decision-making hierarchy that applies in the relevant jurisdiction. The decision-making hierarchy is the specific order in which people close to the patient are 'ranked' to determine who the correct person should be to make medical treatment decisions for the patient.[36] It might, for example, be their spouse, child, parent, sibling, friend or carer.

There is some uncertainty about whether a substitute or default decision-maker can *refuse* medical treatment. They may only be permitted to provide *consent* to medical treatment.

Finally, if a patient does not have an advanced health directive and there is no substitute or default decision-maker available to make decisions for them, then the health provider will need to formally apply to the relevant court or tribunal for a guardian to be appointed for the patient.[37] There must always be someone separate to the patient who, when the patient cannot make decisions, will 'step into their shoes' and make decisions on their behalf.

RIGHTS OF VULNERABLE PATIENTS

Although all patients are vulnerable while they are in the health system, there are some population sectors that are considered to be especially vulnerable.

Patients who lack capacity, including through mental illness

Patients who cannot provide consent to proposed medical treatment due to a temporary incapacity (for example, because they are unconscious or in a coma) are vulnerable simply because they cannot speak or decide for themselves at the time that a decision must be made.

If the situation is an emergency, health providers are permitted to provide medical treatment that is necessary and reasonable in the circumstances.[38] If a patient is wearing a bracelet clearly indicating, for example, that they are a Jehovah's witness and refuse specific treatments or there is some other indicator of their wishes, then health providers should comply with these wishes to the greatest extent possible.

If a patient has prepared a valid advanced health directive then the terms of the directive will apply to the situation. If a patient has not prepared a directive, then a substitute or default decision-maker will need to make the necessary medical care and treatment decisions for the patient.

Patients who are conscious but who lack capacity, such as through mental illness, may still be able to make decisions about their medical care and treatment. The key factor is the ability of the patient to understand the nature and effect of the proposed treatment.[39] In other words, a patient may believe that they are Muhammad Ali, but they may still have the legal right to decide what happens to their body.

For a person to demonstrate sufficient decision-making capacity in relation to health care and treatment, they need to be able to:

- Take in and retain information about their treatment;
- Believe the treatment information; and
- Weigh that information (balance the risks posed by the treatment with their own needs).[40]

If the person is unable to provide consent to medical treatment, then an order from a court or tribunal providing consent for medical treatment will usually be required. The fact that a person lacks capacity does not deny them the protection offered by the law of consent to treatment – it is just that someone else must stand in their shoes to consider all options and make the choice for them.

Patients with language barriers

Patients who have difficulties with the governing language are entitled to have access to an interpreter to assist them in their medical treatment decisions while they receive health care services. Language and similar communication problems do not entitle medical treatment decisions to be made without the person's consent, it simply adds complexity to the provision of medical care to the person concerned.

Elderly patients

Some older people can find it difficult to be assertive and as a result may be too compliant in their health care. It is not uncommon for older people to believe that they will be 'punished' if they cause 'problems', such as by asking too many questions.

There is some evidence of discrimination against the elderly in the area of health care.[41] Elderly people, in general, consume more health services and contribute less to the current economy than younger people. Some health commentators have raised concerns that these pressures could affect how elderly people are treated in the health system and the care options that will be made available to them in the future.[42]

It can also be physically difficult for elderly patients to attend medical centres and hospitals for health care, yet alone to seek second opinions. Home visits are not always available. This is a practical accessibility issue for many older people.

Due to these vulnerabilities, advocacy can be especially important for patients who are older to ensure that medical treatment decisions are being made 'freely and voluntarily'. Families and friends of elderly patients are encouraged to support the patient to express their wishes wherever possible. If this is too stressful for the patient, then they may need someone they trust to uptake this advocacy role on their behalf.

Patients who are minors

Consent for the medical treatment of patients in Australia who are under 18 years of age is generally provided by parents or guardians.[43]

Under the common law, there is provision for minors to consent to medical treatment when they are old and mature enough to have *"...achieved a sufficient understanding and intelligence to enable him or her to understand fully what is proposed."*[44]

Complexity will arise, for example, if a minor consents to medical treatment, but the parent/guardian refuses consent. Or, a minor may seek for their medical treatment to be kept confidential from their parent/guardian. These issues are dependent on the facts in each case and the law that applies in the specific jurisdiction.

RIGHT TO COMPLAIN ABOUT HEALTH CARE

Patients in most jurisdictions have the right to commence and conduct a formal complaint in relation to their health care and treatment should they wish to do so.

CONFIDENTIALITY, PRIVACY AND ACCESS TO HEALTH RECORDS

Although often confused for being the same thing, confidentiality and privacy are in fact very different. Confidentiality is an ethical duty or obligation placed on the shoulders of health providers, whereas privacy is a right of patients that is protected in Australia by both legislation and the common law.

Confidentiality

There is a key ethical requirement that medical practitioners maintain a patient's confidentiality.[45] This stems from the following provision attributed to the Hippocratic Oath:

> Whatever I see or hear in the lives of my patients, whether in connection with my professional practice or not, which ought not to be spoken of outside, I will keep secret, as considering all such things to be private. [46]

Confidentiality is an essential pillar in health care because it encourages people to disclose information that is of a personal nature that they may be uncomfortable revealing if the protection of the duty for confidentiality did not exist. This helps the health provider to treat and care for the patient, as well as the patient who can access better health outcomes through honest communication.

Privacy

Australia has complex legislation in relation to protecting and managing information privacy. Due to the sensitive nature of health information, most jurisdictions treat health information with additional care within their privacy laws.

One of the key areas of the privacy regime concerns access to health information. It is a common (and understandable) misconception that patients own their own health information. This is not the case. Health records are owned by the person who creates the record (for example, the medical practitioner) or the organisation attended by the patient (the clinic, hospital etc.) – not by the person whose information is contained in the health record.

Patients do however have a *right of access* in Australia to their health information.[47] Access to health information can only be lawfully withheld from the person making the request in certain circumstances.

PATIENT RESPONSIBILITIES

Finally, it is important to understand that in addition to their legal rights and entitlements, patients also have responsibilities *to* the health system. Many of these responsibilities are contained in the Charter.

In summary, patients are generally expected to do the following:

- To attend scheduled appointments on time so as not to delay the provision and orderly flow of health service delivery (and to cancel appointments in advance if necessary);

- To pay for health services as directed and agreed in advance and to know what is and is not covered by their private health insurance;
- To respect requirements relating to visiting hours, use of mobile phones, smoking and similar;
- To be responsible in relation to infectious diseases or contagious ailments to minimise the risk of harm to other patients or to health providers;
- To know their health information (medication taken, symptoms and so on) and to give honest and comprehensive health information to health providers to assist in the provision of effective and efficient treatment;
- To speak to health providers about issues of concern (such as if they know that something has been missed or forgotten);
- To give health providers contact information for next-of-kin or substitute decision-makers and to inform them if an advanced health directive exists;
- To treat other patients, visitors, health providers, administrative staff, cleaners and other people with courtesy and respect;
- To respect the privacy of other patients who may be treated in their vicinity;
- To ask questions if they do not understand the health information and treatment options being presented to them;
- To inform the health provider if they have difficulty with language or hearing;
- Inform health providers (as much as possible) if they are unhappy or have an issue with any aspect of their health care or treatment;
- To comply with health treatment that is provided and the instructions that are given;

- To inform health providers if they are receiving health care from any other health providers (including natural or complementary medicine) at the same time;
- To inform health providers of any relevant cultural or religious beliefs that may affect their ability to receive the recommended health care and treatment; and
- To provide a safe environment in their home for visiting health care workers (that are free from smoke, violence, harassment or unrestrained animals).

The responsibility to seek and choose health belongs with the patient. It is not the responsibility of the health system to make someone healthy – only to provide information, advice and treatment at the patient's request.

The right to self-determination that underpins many human rights (which includes the right to refuse medical treatment), is based on the fundamental concept that people are responsible for their own lives. It is the patient's *right and responsibility* to decide whether to accept or refuse advice given to them by a health provider. It is not the responsibility of the health provider to ensure that the patient complies with this advice and acts to become healthy.[48]

CONCLUSION

We hope that the information contained in Chapter 3 and in this Chapter has helped you to build a platform for your own advocacy. It is quite heavy material, but the more you understand the key terminology as well as the policy and legal framework that relates to health care, the more effective you will be as a patient advocate.

In the remainder of this Handbook we will focus on assisting you to develop the specific skills and techniques needed to improve your effectiveness as an advocate, so you feel confident to **negotiate**, **mediate** and/or to **intercede** where required.

KEY LEARNINGS FROM CHAPER 4

- As a patient receiving health services you have rights which are protected by the law.
- Patients must provide consent to any medical treatment they receive. For this consent to be valid, it must be given freely and voluntarily. Patients also require all necessary information and the time to consider that information.
- Patients have the right to refuse medical treatment and to change their mind about whether they consent to or refuse medical treatment at any time.
- Legal rights exist within a practical context that are also influenced by policy and financial factors.

PRACTICE EXERCISE – CHAPTER 4

Stan is 48 years old and a motor mechanic. He purchased his mechanic business from his boss three years ago and has a mortgage as well as a business loan and an overdraft.

Stan has been admitted to a public hospital after suffering an injury and has been told that he needs to have his right hand amputated. Stan's doctor happens to remind him of his niece who lives in New York and is (in his opinion) a bit of a 'silly party girl' so he is struggling to take his doctor seriously. Stan is not married and other than his sister (who also lives overseas) he has no family nearby. He does not have a mobile phone with him in hospital.

Stan decides that he wants a second opinion, if not a third opinion, and expresses this wish to his doctor.

Think about what should happen next. Does Stan get his second opinion? Think about what rights Stan has, how he can exercise these rights and what the likely response/s will be from the staff at the hospital.

This Exercise is designed to help you to think about some of the practical issues that can arise in health care, and how you can use legal and policy rights to get an outcome.

A suggested answer for this Exercise is included at the end of this Handbook.

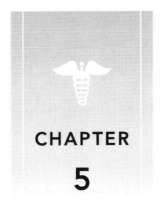

CHAPTER

5

THE IMPORTANCE OF NEUTRALITY

Now that you understand some of the key legal and policy rights that are available to patients in health care, the next step is to learn how to exercise these rights to achieve a specific outcome. This Chapter introduces you to the concept of 'neutrality' and explains how this will become your greatest asset as a patient advocate.

WE ALL WEAR 'SUNGLASSES'

No one else sees the world the same way that you do because no one else has had the same life journey as you have had. We are each heavily influenced by our experiences, environment and heritage. To put it simply, everyone perceives the world through their very own lens (or what we like to call 'sunglasses') – and it is impossible to see the world any other way.

Neutrality is all about being *aware* that this is the case. It is knowing:

- that we are wearing unique 'sunglasses';
- that our sunglasses have a 'tint' (and what this 'tint' actually is); and

- that our perception of a situation is only ever from our perspective.

This means also knowing that our view is inherently limited, and so with a shift in perspective we will be able to see people, problems and solutions entirely differently. This is why neutrality is like your 'secret weapon' – because it can help you to change your life through a change in your perception.

> With neutrality we can see pathways for resolution when others see only conflict. It is what allows us to transcend our own limitations, judgments and opinions to see a new way forward – and this is the most important attribute needed to be an effective patient advocate.

CULTURE, VALUES AND MORALITY IN HEALTH CARE

The most significant 'tints' in our personal sunglasses come from our culture, values and morality. Although these words are often used interchangeably, they each mean very different things which is why we have briefly described each below.

It does not matter how objective we believe we are (or can be), our perception is highly conditioned and influenced by these elements, and so is the perception of the people who work in the health care industry.

Culture

Culture can be defined as *"the customary beliefs, social forms, and material traits of a racial, religious, or social group"* also *"the set of shared attitudes, values, goals, and practices that characterizes an institution or organization."*[49]

A hospital will therefore have its own culture, and this will usually be influenced by the culture of the broader society around that hospital. Patients who share the culture of the hospital will have minimal cultural difficulty during their health journey. However, patients with a different cultural heritage can experience a 'collision'. If this collision is not recognised and understood, then it may lead to conflict and poor health outcomes.

Values

Values can be defined as *"important and lasting beliefs or ideals shared by the members of a culture about what is good or bad and desirable or undesirable. Values have a major influence on a person's behaviour and attitude and serve as broad guidelines in all situations."*[50]

Values highlight the parts of a culture that have significance and are what the culture (collectively) seeks to defend and promote. For example, in Australia there are strong values concerning fairness and access to health care. Whether a patient receives surgery or is entitled to a private room may depend on where they are on a waiting list. This reflects values of fairness, waiting one's turn and due process. Or if one person is in much poorer health than another person, there are values that tell us that the sicker person should receive priority.

Other values include personal privacy (shown through the drawing of a curtain or screen around a patient on a shared ward), visiting hours being restricted (balancing values i.e. the important role of family/friends in health but also the patient's need for rest) and responsible rationing of health resources (shown through a reluctance to carry out futile health tests or treatment).

Morality

Morality tells us what a broader social group perceives as 'right' and 'wrong' or 'good' and 'bad'. It can be defined as *"conformity to ideals of right human conduct"*.[51] It places a value judgment, in effect, on values and culture.

The health system in Australia is significantly influenced by morality. This morality is partially derived from the predominantly Christian religious heritage of many health providers, as well as from the morality that is embedded in the Australian legal system. For example, a woman in Sydney seeking an abortion will be confronted with the legal *and* moral perspective that her request may, depending on the circumstances, be a crime.[52] This is in respect of medical treatment that is viewed very differently in other parts of Australia due to different moral perceptions. Similar moral views exist in relation to a patient's right to refuse medical treatment, particularly if this will result in death, and even more so in relation to euthanasia.

Another example of the impact of values and morality in health care can be seen in the attitudes of some health providers towards patients who, through perceived 'lifestyle choices', have poor health outcomes, such as patients who are smokers or who are obese.[53] According to one study of medical students, approximately 40% of the students surveyed were found to be unconsciously biased against obese people due to a perception that obese people would not follow treatment plans.[54]

WHY NEUTRALITY MATTERS

The role of a patient advocate is to **negotiate**, **mediate** and/ or to **intercede** on behalf of a patient while that person is seeking access to, or is receiving, health services. To do this well, you need the ability to view what is happening to you or to the patient clearer than anyone else can see it – including the patient.

> You need a 'bird's eye view' of the situation from 1000 feet, and for this perspective to be as objective, detached and unemotional as possible.

Neutrality can be defined as *"the quality or state of not supporting either side in an argument, fight war, etc."*[55] Synonyms of neutrality include *disinterestedness, equity, evenhandedness, fairness, impartiality, justice, detachment* and *objectivity.*[56] Antonyms of neutrality include *bias, favour, non-objectivity, one-sidedness, partiality, partisanship and prejudice.*[57]

In our view, neutrality is the most important of all qualities needed for effective patient advocacy. It is what enables you to identify your own perspective – to see the 'sunglasses' you are wearing – and then be able to identify the 'sunglasses' worn by everyone else. This includes the patient as well as the health providers.

It is not realistic, or even possible, to not wear any 'sunglasses', as we must all see the world through some lens or another. The key is to know the lens that you do wear and how influenced (or 'tinted') it is by your own experiences and heritage. Once you can identify your lens and the lens of another party, a **separation** between you and them will start to form. This separation in perspective is essential if you are going to be able to **negotiate**, **mediate** or **intercede**, because this separation is first step towards finding new solutions.

> You need to be able to see the situation more clearly than the patient can, and to be able to think and act to achieve a result that they cannot achieve for themselves. If you and the patient share the same lens, you may as well not be involved!

By way of example, let's consider the case of Ned and Renee. Ned and Renee are both low-income earners who rely on a government pension. Renee is a heavy smoker who has ongoing complications from diabetes. She now requires surgery to remove two toes on her left foot. Ned had a work-related injury several years ago and as a result he carries a lot of hostility towards the health system and doctors in particular, who he believes just *"rip people off so they can buy more Ferraris"*. Ned insists on handling all discussions with Renee's doctor himself because *"he won't take any of their rubbish"*. Renee is happy for Ned to do all the talking. She doesn't want to do anything to upset him because underneath it all, she knows he is just very frightened about her surgery and what it will mean for them.

Dr Jeffries is Renee's surgeon. He has had a very difficult day where a young mother passed away on the operating table due to unforeseen complications. As he approaches Ned and Renee, he looks over Renee's file, sighs to himself and thinks *"here we go again!"* He can see the cigarettes on the bedside table and as he arrives Ned stands up and says *"look here, we've been waiting for over an hour for you. We're not going to put up with treatment like this!"* Dr Jeffries ignores Ned and starts talking to Renee, who won't make eye contact with him because she doesn't want to upset Ned. She refuses to sign any forms or to speak with Dr Jeffries. After waiting in silence for a minute Dr Jeffries shrugs and thinks *"I don't need this today"* and leaves to attend to another patient.

At this point, the relationship between Renee and Dr Jeffries has broken down completely. Renee has not received any information about her upcoming surgery which will now be cancelled due to her refusal to sign the Consent Form. So, what caused this to happen? The issue is a lack of neutrality. Ned's 'sunglasses' were highly prejudiced against doctors and the health system in general. He triggered on his fear of being overpowered from his past experience as well as his insecurity due to his own lack of education. He also wanted to be 'in charge' of Renee because of his deep anxiety for her. Ned has no awareness that his own aggressive stance towards Dr Jeffries caused the issue in the first place.

Dr Jeffries was also wearing 'sunglasses'. As soon as he saw Ned and Renee he formed a judgment about the type of people they were going to be. He didn't like Ned at all because Ned reminded him of his Uncle Joe who was a heavy smoker and drank too much. He was already upset about what had happened earlier in theatre, and to him this was a fairly small and insignificant surgery compared to his other cases. As a result, he allowed himself to lose patience with Ned and Renee and walk away. The outcome was that each side only saw the other (and the situation itself) from one perspective – there was no awareness of any perspective other than their own. This was not a positive outcome for any of the people involved.

About an hour later Ned and Renee's daughter, Tanya, arrived after work. Tanya loves her parents, but she also knows what they can be like. When she finds Ned and Renee she can tell they have had an argument. She listens while Ned explains how he *"stood up to that doctor who was looking down his nose at him and showed him who was boss!"*. Tanya says, *"but Dad – that means Mum isn't having surgery tomorrow and I thought she has a really serious problem?"*. She looks at Renee who nods and starts to cry quietly. Ned decides he needs a cigarette and goes for a walk.

After sitting with her mother for a few minutes, Tanya goes and finds Lisa who is the nurse in charge of the ward. She asks Lisa if she can have a chat and tells her a bit of Ned's history and that both parents are very stressed and that her mum is upset that the surgery is not going ahead. She says *"I know Mum is not the only patient on your ward, but there is an issue and as you know the system better than anyone can you please give me some suggestions on what we can do to fix this?"* After listening to Tanya, Lisa tells her that Dr Jeffries has also had a very difficult day and that he usually is a real joker who makes his patients laugh. She decides to call Dr Jeffries who agrees to come and have another chat with Renee and Ned, but this time Tanya will be there as well.

When Dr Jeffries arrives Tanya greets him, explains how frightened both her parents really are about the surgery and thanks him for his time and support. She then subtly guides the discussion so that Ned is included, but all of her mother's questions are answered. Dr Jeffries is visibly grateful towards Tanya as he had felt bad about how the previous discussion had ended. He re-schedules the surgery and Renee signs the Consent Form. As he leaves, he tells Ned a quick joke. Ned relaxes and thinks to himself *"this guy may be ok after all"*.

This is an example of 'neutrality' in action. Tanya loved both her parents, but she could see how they were contributing to a poor health outcome for Renee. She could understand why

Dr Jeffries might become frustrated so she thought she could help by acting as a discreet facilitator for the discussion. She was able to diffuse the situation by using empathy to make each person feel valued, while she remained focused on the result. She kept herself 'separate' from the perspective of all other parties. **She didn't share 'sunglasses' with anyone else – her focus was 100% on helping her mother to get the surgery she wanted and needed, and this was the result she achieved.** She negotiated and mediated to achieve the outcome.

It is very difficult to achieve complete neutrality when the patient is someone you love and care about – so it is important not to expect this of yourself! In Tanya's case she knew what Ned was like, but she also knew that underneath his bravado was a fear of being overpowered because of what had happened to him in the past. This provided her with the clarity to persist for a solution.

DEVELOPING NEUTRALITY

Neutrality is not easily achieved, and complete neutrality is impossible. Developing neutrality takes time, and is the result of vigilance, observation and being open to continual feedback. Knowing your 'hot spots' and areas of weakness is essential to your advocacy because it means you will be extra careful and vigilant in these areas.

The first step in developing neutrality is to know the level of 'tint' that currently exists in your 'sunglasses', because our biases and preferences can be very subconscious and difficult to identify! If we don't know what 'tints' exist, we don't know what we have to manage in ourselves and in our interactions with others.

At the end of this Chapter we have therefore compiled a list of 'links' and internet search terms for you to explore. We have also highlighted the ones we believe are essential for you to look up and complete. These exercises are invaluable and are highly recommended before you continue any further in this Handbook.

We will also explore neutrality further in Chapter 7 in this Handbook.

KEY LEARNINGS FROM CHAPTER 5

- We are each highly influenced by our culture, values and morality. These, combined with our own experiences, create the 'lens' through which we see the world.
- Neutrality is your greatest asset as a patient advocate, but it is a quality that takes time and effort to develop.
- Neutrality enables you to create separation from the interests, perspectives and pressures of other people (including the patient) so you have the best chance of seeing a new way forward.
- Your beliefs, biases and preferences can be very subtle and unconscious. It is important to question yourself so you can become more aware of your personal 'lens' and how this may impact the outcomes you can achieve for others.

PRACTICE EXERCISES – CHAPTER 5

The following Four Exercises have been obtained from online resources, each of which is acknowledged and referenced below. We are very grateful to the authors of each Exercise for the skill and expertise that has been applied to assist us all to become aware of our own inherent biases, beliefs and perceptions.

If you are interested in this area it is recommended that you do further online research as there are many fantastic tools available to help you.

Please be honest with yourself to gain the maximum benefit from each Exercise.

Exercise 1: 'The Story' (ESSENTIAL)

This activity consists of a simple sentence, and then asks you 11 questions. We strongly recommend that you do this Exercise.

'The Story' is the work of Gerard Puccio, Ph.D., Chair of the International Center for Studies in Creativity at SUNY Buffalo State, USA and can be accessed via the following link:

< http://www.edgef.org/wp-content/uploads/2016/12/Decision-Making-Exercise-The-Cash-Register.pdf >

Alternatively, if you look up in your search engine the words: "a businessman had just turned off the lights" you should be able to find it.

Exercise 2: Project Implicit – Hidden Bias Tests (ESSENTIAL)

Project Implicit was founded in 1998 with the goal of educating the public about implicit social cognition. There are a number of tests you can take including on the topics of age, race and gender. To take these tests please visit:

< https://implicit.harvard.edu/implicit/selectatest.html >

Each test will take approximately 20-30 minutes to complete. It is recommended that you undertake the test in a quiet, distraction-free zone.

Exercise 3: Picking Facts, Opinions, Biases and Stereotypes

This activity involves reading three short paragraphs and seeing if you can identify the facts, opinions, biases and stereotypes included. The activity is provided by Quizlet and is available via the following link:

< https://quizlet.com/213552901/teas-primary-sources-facts-opinions-biases-and-stereotypes-flash-cards/ >

Alternatively, if you look up in your search engine the words: "facts biases stereotypes" you will find some useful resources.

Exercise 4: Four Case Studies

The four cases below are each useful in helping to highlight the values and moral issues that can be triggered in health care.

'Malcom'

Produced by Orr, R, Continuing "'Futile' ICU Support at Relatives' Insistence, The Center For Bioethics & Human Dignity - Trinity International University. Please access via this link: < http://cbhd.org/content/continuing-futile-icu-support-relatives-insistence >

'Mr Chen'

Produced by Santa Clara University, *Markkula Center For Applied Ethics - The Acupuncture Alternative*. Please access via this link:

< http://www.scu.edu/ethics/dialogue/candc/cases/acupuncture.html >

'Mrs Chan'

Produced by Santa Clara University, *Markkula Center For Applied Ethics Cases in Medical Ethics* - Student Led Discussions. Please access via this link:

< http://www.scu.edu/ethics/publications/submitted/cirone/medical-ethics.html >

'The Dancer'

Produced by Santa Clara University, *Markkula Center For Applied Ethics Cases in Medical Ethics* - Student Led Discussions. Please access via this link:

< http://www.scu.edu/ethics/publications/submitted/cirone/medical-ethics.html >

CHAPTER

6

GETTING STARTED (AND MANAGING THE INITIAL CRISIS)

If you are going to act as a patient advocate for someone you care about, then as well as handling the impact of your own 'sunglasses', you also need to maintain a high level of clarity in your advocacy. In addition to giving yourself the best chance of achieving the desired result, this will also help you to navigate the various personal dynamics and relationships that can arise in times of crisis, fear and tension.

TWO CRITICAL QUESTIONS

In Chapter 1 we briefly mentioned 'momentum'. Momentum is one of the key reasons why a person's health care and treatment plan can go off course – sometimes resulting in serious consequences for everyone involved. Taking the time to 'pause' (even if only for a few minutes) enables the cycle to be broken. It can be the difference between feeling like you are in command and feeling like you are on a roller coaster.

> The key is to continually ask yourself
> these two critical questions:
>
> **"Who am I helping?"** and **"What am I here to achieve?"**

It is easy to become distracted, overwhelmed or confused in the health system, so maintaining clarity and focus is essential. If you are the patient, then having clarity and focus on what you wish to achieve will help you to become more targeted and effective in your communication with your health team.

In Chapters 2 to 5 we focused on giving you key foundational information so you can build a platform for your own advocacy. The rest of this Handbook will be very different as we shift focus to providing you with very practical help on *how* to perform the role of a patient advocate. This information is based on our actual experiences so it is our hope that you will be able to avoid some common pitfalls in this area!

STARTING YOUR ADVOCACY

A person who agrees to let you be their patient advocate will usually either feel that they have exhausted their own capacity to find a solution to the issue they are facing, or they are simply unable to handle what is happening to them. They may be emotionally drained, disheartened, very ill or very frightened and so they will be looking to 'pass the baton' on to someone else to take up the battle on their behalf.

This can, in itself, easily manifest into a sense of crisis as everything will feel (and be) very emotionally charged. There will be a sense of intensity and urgency to the situation which immediately brings its own momentum. This initial sense of crisis can cause the advocate to lose both their neutrality and their clarity from the very start.

> This is what you, as a new advocate, need to prepare for from the very beginning – because momentum is the enemy of good advocacy and good decision-making.

For example, a mother may call her son and be in a highly distressed state over a sudden and unexpected health event which will result in surgery the next day. She pours out the story and says that urgent intervention is required because she 'refuses' to have any surgery and is determined to go overseas on a holiday tomorrow as planned. Before he knows it, the son is feeling deeply his mother's trauma, agrees that 'something is not right' and is calling the specialist to 'stop the surgery and sort it out'. At this stage, the son's neutrality as an advocate is already gone.

Although the son is understandably shaken by the distress of his mother, he has not taken the time to 'pause' to work out what should be done. He is already caught in momentum. Although his mother should not have surgery if she does not agree to it, there may be an important reason why the specialist scheduled the surgery for the very next day. He needs to separate his perception of the situation from the perception of his mother, so he can think clearly and work towards the best health outcome for her. By agreeing that 'something is not right' he is already seeing his mother's health situation through the same 'sunglasses' as she is.

> Pausing to break the cycle of momentum
> enables perceptual separation to be created,
> and this is essential to effective advocacy.

Issues can also arise in much less dramatic circumstances. For example, if the patient does not understand the language of the health system, it can be easy for the person acting as their advocate to fall into the trap of speaking on the patient's behalf to their health team. This can then evolve into the advocate starting to make decisions for the patient without their authority. Once again momentum can take hold, and through a perceived time pressure or sense of convenience, the rights of the patient to be informed and the decision maker in their own health care can be subtly eroded.

Continually asking yourself **"who am I helping?"** and **"what am I here to achieve?"** is therefore a key technique to help you to avoid these problems and ensures you remain focused and working in your role as an advocate effectively.

DEFINING THE SCOPE OF YOUR ADVOCACY

As soon as you can, it is essential to clarify the work that you need to do on behalf of the person who is the patient. If you are the patient, then this is about clearly defining the outcome you wish to achieve. We call this 'defining the scope' of your advocacy.

Please consider the following Case Study:

Kate and Rose

Kate called a private patient advocate late one evening about her daughter Rose, aged 12.

Kate is a single mother who lives with Rose in Kalgoorlie, Western Australia. Rose was in a cycling accident a year before and suffered severe injuries. She is now in constant pain and gets violently upset - screaming in agony and on occasion needing to be placed in an isolation ward. She has become suicidal and is losing weight quickly. Kate took Rose to a hospital where she received new medication and was put on a pain management program.

At first Rose seemed to settle, and eventually she was allowed to go home. However, she has recently started having psychotic episodes. Kate thinks it must be a side effect from the new medication. The hospital has told Kate that they believe it is post-traumatic stress.

Kate then learns that the pain management treatment given to Rose in hospital was an overdose. In fact, she was given three times more than the prescribed level. Now that the dosage has been reduced, Rose is suffering from withdrawal symptoms. She now has uncontrollable tremors and was recently rushed back to the local hospital. She is also still having surgery in relation to the original injuries, which requires more drugs which in turn causes more psychotic episodes.

One evening Rose has another episode and vandalises the hospital. Kate can no longer cope. The hospital insists that Kate takes Rose home. Kate refuses, as she knows Rose can be dangerous. The hospital threatens to call the police if Kate doesn't take Rose home. Eventually Rose is escorted from the hospital, however when she sees Kate she hits her across the face and vandalises her car. She was immediately medicated, however the hospital still sent her home. Later that night Rose became violent again and punched Kate and threw furniture around the lounge-room. Kate called 000 and the police came and re-admitted Rose to hospital.

Rose was then placed on another pain management plan, however she is now very fearful of how the hospital is treating her. The hospital is assessing the drugs, but still considers the pain management program to be the best available for Rose. They are saying that there are very limited options to treat this level of pain. Kate has carried out her own research and believes there is only one remedy that will break the pain cycle and avoid Rose's psychotic/allergic reactions. This remedy involves a very strong opiate, and the doctors at the hospital are avoiding it as it is considered to be addictive. The hospital wants Rose to stay on the current pain management plan, even though Kate believes the treatment may be causing the allergic or psychotic reactions.

Kate calls a private patient advocate for help after Rose has had yet another psychotic episode and is about to be discharged into her care late in the evening. Kate has not slept for the past three nights. Kate wants to discuss changing Rose's medication with the advocate.

Response:

The advocate in this case was located in Melbourne, and all work was done by phone. The first decision that the advocate needed to make was 'who is the client?' In this case, the decision was made that Kate was the client. This was based on the fact that Rose was a minor, was heavily under the influence of pain relief medication and was suffering frequent psychotic episodes. However, Rose was capable of expressing her wishes – which included a fear of the local hospital and a deep distrust of the pain management plan that was in place.

The second matter for the advocate to determine was whether or not this was a crisis or emergency situation. The advocate came to the decision that it *was* a crisis situation, as Rose was about to be discharged, was likely (based on past events) to then suffer a further psychotic episode and that Kate would have to manage through this alone.

The third decision for the advocate was to determine the nature of the work that was required to be performed. Kate spoke to the advocate at length about the different medication options for Rose. She was highly agitated on the phone. The advocate listened to Kate's wishes and obtained a fairly comprehensive case history over the telephone. The advocate then told Kate they needed a few minutes to think and hung up the phone. After considering the matter, the advocate called Kate back and recommended that a strategy be adopted to try and take the intensity out of the current situation. Specifically, the advocate proposed to work with the hospital to see if Rose could remain in the hospital that evening (with no further medication being provided) to enable Kate to get some needed sleep. This was an act of 'interceding'. Kate agreed, and the advocate was then able to 'negotiate' with the key hospital staff to achieve this result.

Kate slept well for the first time in many nights and the next morning was calmer and more coherent. Kate and the advocate determined that the key priority was to get a new and independent specialist to review Rose's pain management plan. This then became the 'scope of work' for the advocate, which from then on involved a combination of 'negotiating' and 'mediating'.

Although this Case Study relates to private advocacy and may appear overwhelming, Kate and Rose's situation highlights the complexities that can exist in defining the 'scope' of the advocacy work to be performed, as well as showing how dramatically issues can escalate. In Chapter 8 we will give you a very practical tool to help you to breakdown and manage situations like this.

Although you must always discuss your approach with the person who is the patient, sometimes the patient may not know what help they need! They may just feel disempowered and frightened. There is therefore a fine balance between following the wishes of the patient and considering the outcome that could be in their best interests. These two perspectives are often not the same. This is why it is so important that you maintain your neutrality as much as possible so you can think beyond what is being presented to you, while also being aware (and managing) your own opinions and beliefs about the situation.

In the example earlier of the mother and son, the son needed to focus and think clearly about how to really help his mother who may actually need urgent surgery, even though she was feeling very frightened about what was happening to her and was upset about the disruption to her holiday. In this case, supporting his mother to calm down so she could better understand the situation and the options available to her would be a greater support than just immediately cancelling the surgery. It may well be that with more information and discussion (such as a phone call between the specialist, the son and mother together) the timing for the surgery could be delayed a short while to support the mother to feel more comfortable with the process while still gaining the health outcome sought by the specialist.

In any crisis, your priority should always be to reduce the intensity of the situation (i.e. to lessen the crisis itself) in the safest way for all parties. This may not create a 'perfect' outcome, but it will buy some time to allow the crisis to pass so that clearer thinking can return. It is essential to take as much 'heat' out of the crisis as possible. The substantive issues can then be approached without the relevant parties being in a high state of agitation, fear or reaction.

In the above Case Study, the advocate demonstrated neutrality by deliberately not getting caught in the momentum of the case. They terminated the call with Kate so they could take a few minutes to regain their neutrality and really think about what should happen next before calling back and suggesting a new, and much more stable, way forward.

Sometimes several health issues all happen at the same time! If you are helping someone and this is the situation then it is wise not to assume that they will want you to help them with each issue. Always ask questions because there may be some issues that the other person feels are private and so they may want to handle these themselves. A useful analogy is to imagine two lines of parallel railway tracks. You should always stay within the tracks and focus only on what they want you to do. This is the safest course for both you and for the other person who is the patient.

IF IT ALL GOES WRONG ...

Sometimes, despite your very best efforts, momentum will still take hold and your clarity and neutrality will be lost. If this happens, do not panic! In almost all cases the issue can be corrected through a simple 're-set' by going back to basics, seeing where the neutrality was lost and asking yourself once again: **'who am I helping?'** and **'what am I here to achieve?'**.

You are doing your best in a very intense and stressful situation so please do not be too hard on yourself. Just refocus, regain your clarity and get back to work.

KEY LEARNINGS FROM CHAPTER 6

- You are likely to start working as an advocate for someone you care about when they are in a level of personal crisis.
- It is essential that you separate yourself from the momentum of their crisis as much as possible so you can maintain your neutrality, clarity and focus.
- Asking two simple questions: **'who am I helping?'** and **'what am I here to achieve?'** will greatly assist

you to stay clear and on track despite the turbulence around you.

- If the situation suddenly veers off course, just reset, refocus and get back to work.

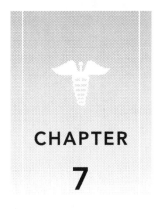

CHAPTER

7

THE FIVE CORE QUALITIES
OF A PATIENT ADVOCATE

The role of a patient advocate is to **negotiate**, **mediate** and **intercede** on behalf of another person to achieve a specific outcome for that person. But how exactly do you negotiate, mediate or intercede? In this Chapter we will introduce you to the five core qualities or personal attributes that you need to be effective in each of these key roles. As you will see, these qualities are also essential 'life skills' that, as you develop and refine them, you will be able to use throughout all areas of your life.

FIVE CORE QUALITIES OF AN EFFECTIVE ADVOCATE

The five core qualities of an effective patient advocate are:

- Assertiveness;
- Empathy;
- Communication;
- Neutrality; and
- Access to Knowledge.

Neutrality is the most important of these qualities and access to knowledge is the least important. In this Chapter we will focus on each of these core qualities in some detail and support you to identify your personal strengths and weaknesses in relation to each one. We will also give you some help should you wish to strengthen your capacity in any of these areas.

Patient advocacy is all about finding your voice and knowing how to use it effectively. These five qualities are all part of this process. Developing these qualities will help you to know when to speak, how to speak, what to say – and also when to listen, so that you have the best chance to achieve the outcome you are seeking.

ASSERTIVENESS

Assertiveness does not mean being bossy! Assertiveness, in the context of patient advocacy, means the capacity to:

- Identify an outcome or result that you want to achieve;
- Identify what you need to do in order to achieve that outcome; and
- Be confident enough to go out and do your best to achieve it, with the minimum level of conflict and disharmony.

For example, it could be that for a patient's health to improve, they need to consult a particular specialist who is not very accessible. Being assertive means knowing that the patient needs to get to this specialist, determining the best way to go about it and then putting that in motion. Having the courage to try, and then pushing past any limitations perceived by people within the health system is all part of being assertive.

Passive, Assertive or Aggressive?

There are three basic operating styles that most people employ at any given moment: assertion, passivity and aggression. Assertion can be confused with 'aggression', but in our view aggression is simply the extreme expression of assertion. This link can be useful if you want to learn more about the differences between these three styles:

< https://www.skillsyouneed.com/ps/assertiveness.html >

Here are three examples of these operating styles applied to some 'everyday' situations:

Example 1: Jill works hard and looks forward to some time for herself when she gets home. However, nearly every evening over the past fortnight her elderly neighbour has popped in for a cup of tea and a chat. Jill values her neighbour's friendship, but does not want this dynamic to continue. How can she tell her neighbour?

- Passive response: "I'll put the kettle on".

- Aggressive response: "Look you've got to stop coming over every evening. Can't you understand that I need some personal time?"

- Assertive response: "I often enjoy having tea with you, but I need a bit of time to myself these days when I get home from work. How about making Tuesday and Thursday afternoons the time when we get together? I'd really like that." Jill can then decide if she wants to phase the visits out even more than this – but it is a harmonious first step in achieving her desired result.

Example 2: Waiting at the pharmacy counter for a prescription, Janet is about to be served when someone behind her says to the pharmacist, *"excuse me, I just have a quick question."* There are many people waiting in line for their prescriptions to be filled. What should she do?

- Passive response: "Well if it's just a quick question, ok, go ahead."

- Aggressive response: "I'm sorry but I've got better things to do than wait here and listen to your problem. Wait your turn."

- Assertive response: "I've been waiting a long time and it's my turn now. I don't expect to be very long either."

Example 3: Jack is attending a medical conference. Jack was introduced earlier to Jane by an acquaintance, however he cannot remember her name. Jane has now joined a conversation Jack is involved in. Jack wants to ask her a question, but doesn't know how to address her, what should he do?

- Passive response: Jack is embarrassed and decides to say nothing and wait until someone else says her name first.

- Aggressive response: Jack says to Jane, "You didn't speak clearly enough earlier, what's your name again?"

- Assertive response: Jack waits until an appropriate break in the conversation and then says "sorry, but I didn't catch your name earlier. I was a bit overwhelmed with names at morning tea. What is it again?" He then uses her name at the first opportunity to help him remember it.

If you are unsure how assertive you actually are, then you can do some online tests to get some objective feedback. We recommend the following test, but if you look up 'assertiveness questionnaire' or 'assertiveness inventory' in your search engine you will find some useful resources:

< http://www.therapymatters.co.uk/files/Assertiveness%20questionnaire.pdf >

Developing Assertiveness

The patient, due to their health situation, is likely to have lost the capacity and energy to assert for themselves. That is why they need your help!

The behaviours of a patient advocate who is assertive would include the following:

- An assertive person believes in himself or herself.
- An assertive person makes it a point to always be well-informed.
- An assertive person is clear about the outcome they want to achieve.
- An assertive person presents in a calm, clear and respectful manner.
- An assertive person actively listens and integrates other people's point of view.
- An assertive person seeks to generate a win-win solution wherever possible.

If you are not naturally assertive, then it is important to develop this attribute as quickly as possible. The following exercises are designed to assist you in the event that you feel it is necessary to strengthen your capacity in this area.

Practice Exercise 1

It can be very hard to come up with the 'right' response when you are under pressure. There isn't much time to think, and you may be feeling strong emotions. It is good to go back and think over any past exchanges with other people in which you felt you were not assertive enough and to consider how you could have responded in a more assertive manner. This may have been with a salesperson, with a friend, with your hairdresser – anyone!

The following questions are designed to help you in this process:

1. For one week, monitor any of the criticisms or negative feedback that you get from other people.
2. Write down each comment and who it was from.
3. Write down your response at the time.
4. Evaluate your response. Was it assertive? Was it negative or defensive? What did you do right?
5. If you were unhappy with your initial response, write a more assertive response that you can use in the future.

Practice Exercise 2

Some people find it difficult to make requests of other people. They may feel that they do not have the right to ask, or they may fear the consequences of asking. This can result in an avoidance in asking for help, even when it is perfectly reasonable to do so.

Think of at least one situation in which your needs, desires, or expectations are not being met, or where you might need help. Think about the situation and how you might use the tips above to assist you. Write how you could go about making a request, and if you feel comfortable, then act upon it.

Practice Exercise 3

It is perfectly reasonable to do favours for others and to take on extra responsibilities when asked. Problems arise, however, if you do this because you cannot say 'no'.

Carry a pen and paper with you for one week. Write down any requests that are asked of you that you don't feel completely comfortable about. Make a note of what you did in the situation. Later, when you have had some time to think, decide whether you are happy with your response. If not, write down a response that you think would have been better. After you've practiced this for a while, try using these skills to say 'no' to requests that you do not wish to take on in the future.

Practice Exercise 4

Start to become aware of people around you who you see as being assertive and observe how they communicate with others. If you hear any good 'assertion phrases' write them down for future reference. It can also be useful to observe how the other person receives and responds to the assertive communication.

You may be pleasantly surprised at how positive these communications can be. If assertiveness is done well, the other person often feels respected and that what is being said is quite reasonable.

Managing Aggression

Some people are on the opposite end of the spectrum and are prone to aggression. This is as much of an issue in patient advocacy as being passive, because you will cause unnecessary conflict and stress within an already stressed and intense environment.

People who are naturally aggressive may have had some powerful life experiences that have 'taught' them that it is necessary to operate in this manner. Indeed, there may be many situations in which their aggression has been effective – but it will not be effective in patient advocacy. You will need to work on changing this behaviour.

Some simple techniques that may help you to convert aggression into assertiveness include:

- Consciously working on being 'kind' to other people. This forces you to consider the other person you are interacting with and how you could express kindness in the situation. You cannot be kind and aggressive at the same time!

- Ask a close friend or family member to provide feedback and support. This will be as uncomfortable for the other party as it will be for you!

- It can help to imagine that you have a volume 'dial', like on a stereo, with numbers from 0 to 10 where the volume can go from mute to full sound depending on the position of the dial. People who are aggressive may continually be at volume level 8 or 10. Similarly, people who are naturally passive may have a dial that is often at 1 or 2. Consciously work on turning the volume level to 5 or 6.

- Be aware of the response from other people and use these responses as a gauge of the effectiveness of your communication. Positive feedback is a wonderful incentive and tells you that you are making progress!

Making a Change

Do not expect to become assertive overnight! It takes time to learn these new skills and to apply them consistently. If you have established patterns towards either passivity or aggression you may also require some external support and encouragement to build the quality of assertiveness within yourself. Be patient!

It may also take time for other people around you to adjust to your new operating style. If you used to be quite aggressive, people around you will most likely respond positively to the shift to assertiveness because they will appreciate the softening in your manner. However, if you were more passive, some people may respond negatively to your new assertiveness, as they may feel threatened when you start to act (in their view) more 'strongly'. This doesn't mean you are wrong! They are simply adjusting to the change. This is natural, so it is important not to be thrown off course.

EMPATHY

In order for you to achieve an improved health outcome for a patient, the patient must feel that they can trust you and that you are 'with them' on their health journey. This requires empathy.

Empathy can be defined as *"the ability to imagine oneself in another's place and understand the other's feelings, desires, ideas and actions."*[58] In other words, empathy is the ability to walk in another person's shoes.

There is often confusion between empathy and sympathy. Empathy and sympathy are very different in their emotional meaning and level of power in interpersonal relationships. Empathy has been described as the ability to mutually experience the thoughts, emotions and direct experiences of others.[59] Empathy expresses the notion that *"I understand how you feel right now"*. If Fred says to Jenny *"you must be angry about what he just said to you!"*, this is a statement of empathy because Fred is expressing his own experience of what Jenny is feeling based on what he overheard. He is sharing it with her.

Sympathy is a feeling of recognition of another's suffering, but there is no personal 'melding' with the other. For this reason, empathy is often considered the deeper emotional experience and creates the better relationship or bond. An example of a 'sympathy statement' is when Betty says, *"Carol, I'm really sorry about your husband's accident."* Betty is expressing her feelings about Carol's husband's situation and is being considerate and kind, but she is not as personally or deeply involved.

An empathetic statement is often described as having a 'you' statement, such as *"you must be feeling..."*, whereas a sympathy statement often begins with an 'I' declaration – it is more *"how I feel about [you, this or that]"*.

Using Empathy

Empathy is a very powerful tool. It can help to build a close and rewarding bond with the person you are helping by revealing their true needs or fears, it can create genuine opportunities when dealing with health providers and it can de-escalate contentious situations. In the example of Ned and Renee from Chapter 5, Tanya actively used empathy to create the result she knew her mother wanted achieved.

When using empathy it is important to be genuine, as people can often tell when someone is not being sincere in their use of empathy. If empathy is not used carefully and sincerely, the other person may feel patronised which will create the opposite result to what is intended.

It is a fine line between using empathy to build trust, and using empathy to manipulate another.[60] Using empathy as a technique for manipulation is not in itself 'positive' or 'negative', as this will depend on the context and the motivation. In these cases, the empathy may not be as 'genuine', but it can still be appropriate and effective. The onus is on the advocate to be aware of what they are doing and why they are doing it, and to be as responsible as possible.

There is also a significant connection between empathy and neutrality.[61] In the earlier example Tanya maintained her own neutrality. She did not express judgment or disapproval towards either of her parents or Dr Jeffries: her focus was to de-escalate the conflict so her mother could have the surgery she needed. This is how empathy and neutrality can be used effectively *in combination.*

> Neutrality will enable you to see a way forward,
> and empathy will assist you in getting people
> to 'buy in' to your proposed solution.

Example phrases you may find useful include:

- "Thank you again for giving me some time – I can see how busy you are. I just need to know the best way to contact Dr Smith?"

- "OK Doctor, I believe I understand but it is quite overwhelming for me – so you really feel this is the best way for me to go? Thank you for being so clear with me. If I wanted to speak to another doctor - just for my own peace of mind - how would I best arrange this?"

- "Hi - are you the nurse in charge? I can see you are really on the run today – is it best for me to make an appointment to discuss two or three quick issues with you about my dad's treatment? It doesn't have to be now – just sometime today would be perfect."

- "I understand your advice – my concern is that this outcome is exactly what my sister has really been dreading. She cries whenever it comes us, so it's going to be a huge shock for her. Can we brainstorm this together to see what other treatments are available? Let's just put everything on the table..."

- "Excuse me, I know you are really short-staffed today – unfortunately my husband hasn't received his dinner yet and I think it's been missed. Is there someone I can call to arrange some food? He's a diabetic so missing a meal will cause him big issues."

How to Develop Empathy

If you are unsure how empathetic you actually are, then you can do some online tests to get some objective feedback. For example:

< https://greatergood.berkeley.edu/quizzes/take_quiz/empathy > or

< https://psychology-tools.com/test/empathy-quotient >

You can also look up 'empathy tests' or 'am I empathetic?' in your search engine to find other useful resources.

Learning to show empathy is an acquired skill, which takes time to develop. Some common and practical techniques that can help you in this area include:[62]

1. Listen closely to what the other person is saying. This will help you to absorb what they say and respond

appropriately. Remove any distractions (for example, put away your phone). Focus all your attention on what the other person is saying.

2. Pay attention to the words the other person says, but also to the way these words are communicated, including voice inflection, tone and mannerisms.

3. Let your non-verbal cues convey your interest in the person. Be aware of your body language. Do not fidget or act in a manner that may indicate disinterest. Direct 100% of your attention towards them.

4. Reflect back what the other person just said. This helps to show that you are listening, understanding and interpreting what they have said. This also provides them with the chance to elaborate further on what is being expressed and demonstrates your concern. For example: *"I am so sorry to hear that you received a negative test result - I can see this is very hard for you to talk about"*. It is important to remember to focus on how the *other* person is feeling and not on how you feel about their circumstances.

5. Validate the other person's emotions. This helps to convey your acceptance and respect for their feelings. For example: *"I can understand why you would be so upset"* or *"anyone would find this difficult"* or *"your reaction is totally normal"*.

6. Offer personal support. Offering personal support goes beyond words to let the other person know that you genuinely want to help them. For example: *"I want to help in any way I can, so please let me know what I can do to help."* Once again, it is important to be sincere.

Below is another Practice Exercise that may assist you in developing this skill:

Practice Exercise: 'Checking In'

A very simple exercise is to 'check in' with someone else to see whether or not you can identify the correct, or at least the closest, emotion to what that person is feeling at any given time.

Try to determine what emotion the other person is feeling, and then ask the other person to see if you are correct. You can check in by using a question or a statement, for example:

- You look a bit anxious right now
- You're looking like you've won the lottery!
- You seem like you're in a fair bit of pain
- Are you worried about something?

Managing Over-Involvement

It is possible to go too far in your level of empathy. Although this is natural considering the relationship between you and the patient, it will make it very difficult for you to maintain your neutrality. You may not be able to separate and hold your own 'sunglasses' and as a result you can easily become caught in the perspective of the patient.

If you become aware that a situation of 'excessive empathy' has occurred, you will need to 're-set' yourself in a safe and responsible manner. It is not fair or appropriate to suddenly become cool towards the other person, as they will not understand what has happened. Just gradually regather your own neutrality. In order words: put your own 'sunglasses' back on!

COMMUNICATION

Effective communication, in the context of patient advocacy, is 'two ways' – there must be effective communication from you *towards* the patient and health providers, but you must also be able to listen and absorb the communication *from* others.

What is Communication?

Communication can be defined as *"the imparting or exchanging of information by speaking, writing or using some other medium."*[63] The act of communication is generally considered to involve verbal, non-verbal, and para-verbal components,[64] specifically:

Verbal Communication

Verbal communication refers to the actual words that are spoken. Words that are critical or judgmental will almost always result in 'doors closing' as the listener will become defensive.[65] If, however, you can use words that are more positive and that make 'OK' an issue or a problem (as much as is possible), it can result in 'doors opening'. In other words: try not to make anyone 'wrong'. Focus on solutions.

It is also important to be efficient and targeted in verbal communication. Lengthy and detailed speech can be confusing to the listener, it may cause irritation (due to a perceived wastage of time) and your message may also lose its impact.[66]

Non-Verbal Communication

Non-verbal communication is extremely powerful. Common non-verbal cues include facial expressions and body language.[67] For example, gathering up your papers can signal a desire to end the conversation, while checking a mobile phone while someone is speaking can convey disinterest. Be very aware of your non-verbal cues at all times!

Para-verbal Communication

Para-verbal communication is *how* we say something, not *what* we say.[68] It includes the tone, pitch, and pacing of your voice. A sentence can convey entirely different meanings depending on the emphasis on words and the tone of your voice. Windle and Warren use the very simple and effective example: "*I didn't say you were stupid*", which has six different meanings depending on which word is emphasised.[69]

Windle and Warren explain that when a person is angry or excited, their speech tends to become more rapid and higher pitched. When a person is bored or feeling 'down', their speech tends to slow and take on a monotone quality. When a person is feeling defensive, their speech is often abrupt.[70] Being aware of these signals in communication, as well as within your own communication, can provide you with some important cues to guide you in your advocacy.

> These techniques can help you to 'change course', even in the middle of a sentence, if you suddenly detect that the other party is not responding in the way you want them to respond. You may only have one chance at conveying your message, so these communication cues are very important!

The Importance of Listening

Being a good communicator requires you to be as effective in listening as you are in speaking. Sometimes what a person *says* is the issue is not the real issue at all! Effective listening will be necessary to truly determine the nature of the problem and how you can help.

Listening is a combination of hearing what another person says, and psychological involvement with the person who is speaking.[71] Listening requires more than hearing the words – it requires a desire to understand another person, an attitude of respect and acceptance, and a willingness to try and see an issue from another person's point of view.[72] Genuine listening therefore also requires a high level of concentration![73]

Styles of Communication

People generally prefer one of the following four communication styles: passive, passive aggressive, assertive and aggressive,[74] as shown below:

- Passive communication: *"Oh, it's nothing, really..."* or *"You choose, anything is fine."*

- Passive-aggressive communication: *"Why don't you go ahead and do it, my ideas aren't very good anyway ... you always know better in any case".*

- Assertive communication: *"Can you please move your car? I am late for an appointment but can't get out of the garage,"* and *"I am so sorry, but I won't be able to cook dinner tonight as I have a last-minute project to complete."*

- Aggressive communication: *"No, I've decided I'm going to do this my way."*

How to Become a Better Communicator

If you are unsure about your own communication style, then you can do some online tests to get some objective feedback. For example:

< https://www.mindtools.com/pages/article/newCS_99.htm >

< https://www.glassdoor.com/blog/quiz-whats-your-communication-style/ > or

You can also look up 'communication styles' or 'am I good communicator?' in your search engine to find other useful resources.

For the purpose of patient advocacy, an assertive communication style is considered optimal. To assist you in developing this style, the following is recommended:[75]

1. *Body Language:* Do not shy away from the person with whom you are speaking. Maintain a relaxed posture regardless whether you are the one speaking or listening.

2. *Speech and Attentiveness:* When speaking, be clear and concise. Speak on important matters directly and do not waste time. Make sure you ask whether or not they understand what you are saying, and be willing to further explain any of your points. Do not expect someone to just 'know' what you are saying (even if it is crystal clear in your own mind!)

3. *Patience:* During your communications with others always give them time to communicate their issues as well. This is particularly important if you lean towards an aggressive style of communication. Remaining focused on what they are trying to communicate will show them that you are open to their point of view. If you are confused as to what someone may be requesting, then repeat back to him or her what you think they said and ask if that is correct. Often this will inspire the speaker to be clearer and more specific about their needs.

4. *Be pleasant:* Practice being pleasant. For example, smile when you deliver your message. Even if you speak over the phone, the other person can 'hear' your smile. Practice basic etiquette, such as acknowledging the other person, listening to both the verbal and non-verbal cues, and generally being polite. This alone can make a tremendous difference to the effectiveness of your communication!

5. *Relax:* If your emotions can sometimes get in the way of delivering your message, practice relaxation methods such as deep breathing, distraction, and meditation to help you to maintain your composure.

The following two techniques may also be useful in helping you to improve the effectiveness and success of your communication:

Reflective Listening

Reflective listening is the process of restating, in your own words, the feelings and/or message that has been expressed. By reflecting back to the speaker what you believe and understand, you validate that person by giving them the experience of being heard and acknowledged.[76] You also provide an opportunity for the speaker to give you feedback about the accuracy of your perceptions, thereby increasing the effectiveness of your overall communication.[77] The following four techniques may also assist you in developing this skill:[78]

1. *Paraphrasing:* A brief, succinct statement reflecting the content of the speaker's message, for example, *"what I am hearing is that you believe David needs intensive physiotherapy if he is to have any chance of being able to return and live independently, is this correct?"*

2. *Reflecting:* A statement that conveys understanding of the feeling that the listener has heard, such as *"to me it seems that you are very worried about David's ability to actually do the exercises given, is this right?"*

3. *Summarising:* A re-statement of the main ideas and feelings of the conversation to show your understanding. For example: *"so to clarify, it seems to me that you are very worried about David and are concerned about his declining mental health - especially if he isn't able to see some progress in his rehabilitation soon".*

4. *Questioning:* Asking open questions to gain information, encourage the speaker to tell their story, and gain clarification. For example: *"I'm confused, are you worried that David may actually try to discharge himself from hospital, or is there something else that is worrying you?"*

The 7C's

The 7C's of effective communication were first published in 1952 and remain well regarded today.[79] According to Cutlip and Center, the 7C's refer to communication that is: complete, concise, concrete, considered, courteous, clear and correct.[80] For example:

1. *Complete:* In a complete message, you have given the listener everything they need to be informed and be able to act (if needed).

2. *Concise:* When you're concise in your communication, you keep to the point and keep it brief.

3. *Concrete:* When your message is concrete, then your listener has a clear picture of what you're telling them.

4. *Considered:* When your communication is considered, you have taken into account the other person's opinions, knowledge, mindset and background. You relate to the recipient.

5. *Courteous:* Courteous communication is friendly, open, and honest.

6. *Clear:* When writing or speaking to someone, think about your goal or message. What is your purpose in communicating with this person? If you're not sure, then the other person won't be sure either!

7. *Correct:* When your communication is correct, it fits the other person. Correct communication is also accurate communication.

NEUTRALITY

Neutrality, in the context of patient advocacy, was introduced in Chapter 5. Neutrality means an advocate is aware of the 'sunglasses' they are wearing and the potential effect of their lens on the situation before them.

Developing Your Neutrality

As introduced in Chapter 5, the first step in developing neutrality is to know the areas in which you may *not* be neutral. These are your personal 'hot spots', and can include:

- Your history with the patient, family or friends;

- Your previous experience in the health system and whether this has made you either 'pro' the system (resulting in a tendency to accept the limitations of the system) or 'anti' the system (resulting in a negative perspective in which the system is 'wrong' and 'must be changed'). This can extend to views like *"all doctors are arrogant"* or *"nurses never rock the boat"*, or *"all nurses are wonderful"* or *"XYZ hospital is fantastic"* and so on, all of which means that 'fresh' eyes are not being applied to what is happening *right now*;

- Your personal biases or triggers. These do not need to be confined to race, sexuality or gender. They can also relate to general approaches to life. For example, you:

  ➢ may not like 'messy' life situations or people;

  ➢ may 'judge' people who are on government benefits;

> ➤ may have issues with authority figures or people who you see as arrogant;

> ➤ may be jealous of wealthy surgeons;

> ➤ may not like people who do not have good social manners;

> ➤ may have problems with people who don't maintain personal hygiene;

> ➤ may have strong personal views around topics such as euthanasia, age of consent to medical treatment and similar, which can result in you projecting your values on other people.

Any area that triggers a feeling of intensity or an emotional reaction within you is a 'hot spot' for you and therefore an area where your neutrality could be affected.

Remaining Vigilant

Maintaining neutrality requires awareness. It does not necessarily require 'positive action' in the same way that assertiveness, empathy and communication may require action. Maintaining neutrality requires constant vigilance and attending to issues as and when they arise.

Following are some keys to assist you in maintaining neutrality:

- Be aware of momentum. Always take the time necessary to 'pause' from a situation so you can ask yourself whether you are being rushed or are triggered by what is before you. If so, remind yourself of the greater objective or task at hand. It can also be useful to review your notes to see if anything has been missed that could be relevant.

- Develop a checklist. Ask yourself:

    1. What is my potential 'Achilles Heel'? Where could I get caught? Could I become:
        - Overly sensitive?
        - Too passive?
        - Too aggressive?
        - Over-promising?
        - Too involved in the "pain"/emotion of the situation?
        - Am I projecting my own success or failure cycle?
        - Am I (unduly) triggering on any aspect of this situation?

    2. How clear has my communication been? Have I listened well? Has everyone understood my communication?

    3. Is the story I'm being told the whole 'truth'? Is there another side to this issue? If so, what might that be? Consciously considering the other available perspectives is a very useful technique for maintaining neutrality.

Neutrality and Empathy

As noted briefly above in relation to empathy, the qualities of neutrality and empathy work very effectively together.

Neutrality does not mean being 'cold'. It just means maintaining a sense of detachment and 'separateness' so you can view the situation as clearly as possible at all times. Neutrality is about having awareness that there are always two sides to an issue. Empathy can be of tremendous assistance in bringing these two perspectives closer together. However, without neutrality, you will not be able to see that these different 'sides' or perspectives even exist in the first place.

ACCESS TO KNOWLEDGE

You do not need to be an 'expert' on the health system to be able to help someone else. In fact, specialised knowledge can be a limitation as it can create conscious and subconscious 'beliefs' about what is or isn't possible in the health system.

Your task is to help someone with a specific issue. This requires you to be able to determine the nature of the problem and develop a strategy to resolve that problem. Not having 'industry knowledge' can mean that you will have a more open mind and can seek solutions that may not normally be considered possible. In other words, the absence of knowledge can open the door for a new creative solution.

Some knowledge will however be required, and this knowledge may come from 'within' you (that is, from your own experience), from external sources, or from a combination of both.

Managing Your Internal Knowledge

The first step is to do an 'internal audit' to ascertain what knowledge you already possess about the current situation. It is not 'right' or 'wrong' that you have internal knowledge, what matters is that you are aware of the knowledge that you possess. For example, you may have been to every medical appointment with your elderly father for the past three years. This is very powerful knowledge!

The next step is to assess the quality of your knowledge. Is your knowledge from a narrow or wide pool or field of study? Has the industry or sector changed since you last were involved in that field? Who did you obtain your knowledge from? Is this a reputable source? Are you viewing your knowledge through 'tinted' 'sunglasses'?

These are difficult questions, and it is very hard to 'qualify' your own knowledge, but it is important to try to ensure that the best possible knowledge is underpinning the advocacy that you are seeking to provide.

Gaining Knowledge from External Sources

Do not worry if you do not immediately have the knowledge required to resolve the current problem. Provided you know what knowledge you require, it is almost always possible to find out the information you need.

Following are some suggested techniques to assist you in this situation:

- Think about who is the 'best' doctor, specialist, hospital or organisation in relation to the patient's situation within the patient's area. Is there a 'peak body'? If so, then contact the organisation or person and ask for advice on who or where the patient should go as a 'starting point'.

- Do some research on the Internet and read some journal articles. Once certain names, hospitals or facilities start to 'repeat' in what you are reading, it may indicate that it could be another starting point for advice and information.

- If it seems that resources or options are limited within your local area, then it may be necessary to explore options in another location.

- Think about who you already know, or who you may know who may know someone else. Exhaust all your own avenues for assistance.

Regardless of the source of the information, you still need to be discerning about the quality, relevance and appropriateness of what you learn.

It is also important not to 'read in' information that is not there when researching and seeking access to knowledge. 'The Story' Exercise in Chapter 5 aimed to show how easy it can be to 'read in' information that doesn't exist! This can apply very easily to research. You need to be careful not to 'read in' details or solutions that you *want* to see, and ensure you are only reading and learning about what is relevant and applicable for the patient – good and bad.

CONCLUSION

This Chapter is very comprehensive as it aims to give you practical support to develop the attributes and qualities that you may need to be able to speak up and help someone you care about while they are within the health system. You may need to return to this Chapter several times while you build your understanding and capacity within each area – so please be patient while you are developing these new skills!

KEY LEARNINGS FROM CHAPTER 7

- There are five core qualities that you need to develop or refine if you are to be effective as a patient advocate: assertiveness, empathy, communication, neutrality and access to knowledge.
- Neutrality is the most important of these qualities to develop in advocacy, and access to knowledge is the least important quality.
- These qualities are all essential life-skills, so they can be applied throughout all areas of your life.
- If you feel you can improve in any of these areas it is important to do the work, but also to be patient. Developing new ways of behaving takes time!

CHAPTER

8

TAKING ACTION: A FRAMEWORK FOR YOUR ADVOCACY

This Chapter focuses on what you should actually *do* if you are acting as an advocate for someone you care about. You now are aware that you have some legal and policy rights which you can seek to enforce, and you also understand the personal skills, qualities and attributes you need to cultivate within yourself to be effective – so the next step is understanding what you should actually *do* in order to get a result.

As every person's health journey is unique, we cannot give you specific advice for the situation you are facing. However, what we *can* do is give you a step-by-step framework that you can follow which will help you to get from Point A to Point B, and then from Point B to Point C and so on. We have derived this framework from reviewing all of our past cases (in the health area and in the legal area) so we are confident that if you follow each step you will be able to identify the next action to take and how best to take it – until you feel that the best outcome that is available in your circumstances has been achieved.

YOU ARE DRIVING THE CAR

If you are helping someone you care about while they are receiving health care, then this will be because they don't feel they are able to handle everything themselves. They are in need of help and support. If they have agreed (or you have needed) to take on this role, then this means you are 'in charge', providing you are acting in accordance with their wishes.

To put it another way: they need you to take over the wheel and to drive the car to reach the destination – ideally in the fastest time and with the least amount of traffic, bumps and road blocks along the way that is possible.

The first step in acting as a patient advocate is therefore for you to accept that this is now the dynamic and that you are *expected* to pick up the keys, know the destination, select your preferred route, start the car and drive! If you keep thinking the patient is going to take over the wheel you will hesitate and second guess yourself. The patient is of course allowed to change their mind and start managing things for themselves, but until they ask for this, the best support you can give them is to pick up the keys, get into the car and start driving!

WHERE ARE WE STARTING FROM?

The next task is to understand the 'starting position'. This means understanding the health journey that the patient has already experienced, as well as the aspects of their personal history that could impact upon their health care and treatment options.

For example, a friend who has suffered domestic violence over a period of time may not be as able to question a treating doctor as someone who has not experienced personal violence. If you are helping her as her advocate, you need to be aware of this history otherwise you could accidentally make the situation worse by expecting her to 'stand up for herself'. She may not be able to do this, which is why she asked you to help her in the first place!

Alternatively, a patient may have been cycling through the medical system for many years and have lost any sense of hope that a better health outcome could be possible. This will require you to have empathy and to work softly to build hope for a new outcome, as otherwise the patient may reject every solution you propose out of fear – simply because they cannot cope with further disappointment.

Finally, a patient may just be too unwell or frail to handle any change in their treatment or to formulate a strategy. They could also be dependent on a specific medication or person in their health care. In these cases, it may be wiser to keep the patient's care stable and consistent while you assist them to recover their strength before introducing the potential for any change to their treatment plan.

WHERE ARE WE GOING?

The next step is to work out the patient's ideal or preferred destination **as well as** their 'worst case' destination. These are your initial parameters. To give an example, if a patient has an issue with their right hand, their 'preferred destination' might be physiotherapy and if needed minor surgery to solve the issue, and their 'worst case destination' would be amputation of the hand. This is the outcome the patient wants and the outcome they *do not* want.

Knowing these parameters then guides the next action you will take: specifically, should you **negotiate**, **mediate** or **intercede**? If the patient is being wheeled off to surgery for amputation because they were frightened and signed a consent form but didn't really agree to the surgery, then your action is to **intercede**. If there are competing medical opinions about what should happen, then you may need to **mediate** to try and find a new way forward.

This may seem like common sense, however the health system can be very reactive. One opinion or conclusion can quickly lead to another, and before you know it amputation may be seen as the only viable option. Being very clear that this is NOT where the patient wants to go will help you to stop the momentum before it builds and to refocus the health team on ALL other potential options if this is not occurring.

Sometimes you will not be able to achieve the patient's preferred outcome and sometimes the worst case outcome is the outcome that happens. You are not 'all powerful' and neither is the patient's health team. Health is health, and unfortunately sometimes the only option before you will be the one the patient does not want. There is very little that you can do in this situation, other than manage what you can as best you can. If the 'worst case' scenario for the patient is assisted or artificial respiration, then discussing an advanced health directive (if legally available) with the patient may help them to feel that their 'nightmare' will not happen. This may be all you can do.

In other situations, you will not be able to go very far ahead because the patient's situation is complicated due to multiple health issues occurring at the same time. If this happens, your task is to identify the immediate preferred destination and work towards that. This could be finding out more facts. It could be arranging a second opinion. It could be changing hospitals. You may not be able to determine the patient's preferred destination until other pieces in the puzzle have fallen into place. Once again all you can do is handle what is immediately before you, one step at a time, and focus on handling each step to the very best of your ability. For example:

> Sophia contacted a private patient advocate for assistance with her mother. Her mother was Italian, did not speak English, had multiple health conditions and depended entirely on Sophia to manage her health treatment as well as to provide direct care. Sophia had three children and a full-time job. The stress of managing her mother's health needs was causing Sophia to lose sleep and become increasingly anxious. When she contacted the advocate, Sophia was almost hysterical. She did not know what help she needed, only that *she* needed help to prevent herself from becoming unwell as a result of the stress she was experiencing.

> The advocate spent considerable time discussing Sophia's situation and her mother's needs. Over the course of the conversation it became clear that Sophia needed a strategy to lessen her mother's personal reliance upon her. This required engaging different professional and support services for her mother. Reducing Sophia's responsibilities was the 'optimal

outcome' to be achieved. As the case was quite complex, it was agreed to break the case into stages and to tackle each issue one at a time.

Due to Sophia's level of stress and exhaustion, it was determined that the first priority was to engage a private nurse, who spoke Italian, to take on some of the direct caring functions that Sophia's mother required. Once this had been achieved, Sophia and the advocate could discuss the second stage of the strategy, which was to locate a general practitioner who spoke Italian who could coordinate Sophia's mother's treatments and medication. This work became the focus of the second stage of the advocacy.

Breaking the situation down into stages like this can help both you and the patient to develop a sense of empowerment and stability. Taking the time to pause and ask yourself '**where are we going?**' will help you to remain neutral, in the driver's seat and will ensure that short-term decisions are always made with the patient's longer-term and preferred outcome in mind.

WHERE COULD WE GO?

A slight variation to the question '**where are we going?**' is to ask '**where *could* we go?**' Once again this requires you to have the quality of neutrality.

Sometimes people are so burdened by pain or trauma that they lose hope that it will ever end or that life could ever be any better than it is now. This is where you can be a tremendous support to someone you care about. Can a 'cycle' of poor health be stopped or slowed down? Is there an outcome that would create a more holistic health result? Does the patient have an interest or passion that they wish to pursue that could help their recovery or give them some enjoyment? For example:

> Jeanette was an artist who had developed breast cancer. Her ability to paint was a core part of her life, and for Jeanette a life in which she couldn't paint was a life she couldn't contemplate living. When she was diagnosed, her doctor told her that she must focus all her energy on fighting the disease and conserving her strength. Jeanette became very depressed as the side-effects from the medication began to impact her painting.
>
> A friend decided to come with Jeanette to her next medical appointment because she was becoming increasingly concerned about Jeanette's declining state of mind. The friend raised Jeanette's art with her doctor (who hadn't known Jeanette was an artist) and the three of them then worked together on exploring different treatments and medications to ensure any side-effects that affected Jeanette's ability to paint were minimised.
>
> Jeanette was very grateful to her friend for coming along to the appointment because she hadn't realised that a solution that helped her to continue painting was even possible. She started to feel more positive about her future.

It is very common for patients not to know their 'preferred outcome'. They may be so used to the health system, or be so unwell, that they cannot stretch their mind to consider what other solutions could be possible. They may not be able to imagine a life where they feel 'healthy' ever again.

Your neutrality and empathy is what will support the patient in these times. Specifically, understanding them as a person, including *what they would be doing if they were not unwell*, and including this in their treatment plan wherever you can, may be the most powerful support you will provide.

CREATING 'ALLIES'

Once you know the next step in the journey towards the patient's preferred destination, you need to create some 'key allies' to support you in this process.

This requires (once again) you developing and using the qualities of *neutrality* (identifying the allies you need), *empathy* (engaging them so they wish to support what you are doing), *communication* (being able to convey your message in the way you want it heard) and *assertiveness* (being able to get their focus and attention). Access to knowledge may or may not be relevant depending on the situation.

Specifically, you may need to get the rest of the patient's family to support the approach you are taking so you can present to the health team as a 'united front'. You may need to get the support of the treating doctor or specialist. It might be working with the nursing staff to achieve some specific changes in how the patient receives their care. These alliances may relate to 'bigger issues' (like treatment plans, medications and similar decisions) or to 'smaller issues' (like having the family dog brought in to visit the patient, changing the meal plan or having flowers in the room).

Wherever possible, your goal is to create positive relationships as much as you can to help facilitate achieving the desired outcome in the easiest and most harmonious manner possible.

REPAIRING EXISTING RELATIONSHIPS

Sometimes the relationship between a patient and their health provider can break down due to a series of miscommunications or after too many unmet expectations. A patient can feel that they are not being heard (particularly if the provider appears rushed or distracted), and form the view that they are not receiving proper care. Conversely, a health provider can feel that a patient is determined to only hear what they want to hear, or become frustrated when important information is withheld from them. They can then form the view that the patient is being difficult or even obstructive.

You can be a powerful mediator to assist both sides to listen to one another and to create a bridge that rebuilds the relationship. In particular, you can:

- Listen carefully to the patient to identify the specific issues or problems they have. Ask the patient what they would like to see happen in order for the relationship to get back on track. Sometimes this is an apology for miscommunication. Sometimes it is just to feel that they are being listened to and taken seriously. Ask the patient to be honest about whether they really will, or can, give the provider a second chance.

- With the patient's agreement, meet privately with the provider to convey the concerns of the patient. Use your skills to ensure the provider does not feel attacked or that they are being made 'wrong', but rather learns what they can do to improve the relationship.

A non-threatening approach using empathy is always more effective than confrontation.

- Emphasise that your role is not to get in the way, but to help. Some providers can feel reassured that a third party is assisting to get a message to the patient if the relationship breakdown has prevented this from occurring.

- Be assertive and, if necessary, inform them that if the relationship does not improve, the patient will need to explore other options and may not be willing to consent to treatment. Be careful not to directly interfere with medical treatment, but to stress that the patient is having trouble given the breakdown in trust in the relationship. Always avoid burning any of the patient's bridges with their health providers!

- If the situation allows, set small and achievable goals with the patient that you are optimistic can be achieved, so they feel that things are improving. This may help them to develop trust on larger matters.

- If the situation does not improve and the patient is in a hospital, consider involving the Patient Representative. This may assist the issue to be taken more seriously.

If repairing a key relationship is not achievable, then it may be necessary to assist the patient to find new health providers and to then focus on building a positive working relationship with these new providers from the beginning.

NEGOTIATE, MEDIATE, INTERCEDE

Throughout this Handbook we have continually referred to the three key roles of a patient advocate – **negotiate**, **mediate** and **intercede**. In Chapter 2 we provided you with an initial understanding of these roles, however we now wish to address each of these in further depth and to show you how the work you have just done in Chapter 7 is so fundamental to the performance of each of these roles.

It is not uncommon that an advocate will need to perform each of these three roles at the same time (i.e. within the same conversation or series of conversations). You may start a conversation by **interceding**. This means you take an action (i.e. by speaking) to create a wedge to stop, slow down or change the direction of a current course of treatment. The level of intensity or drama attached to interceding will depend on the *timing* of your action. Obviously interceding while someone is being wheeled down the corridor towards theatre is much more dramatic for everyone involved than interceding three days before the surgery. Wherever possible, aim for your interceding to be as low impact as possible – but if a patient has consented to surgery and then changes their mind you may have no choice but to be 'dramatic' and intercede at quite a late stage.

Negotiating is all about finding your way forward. It may be convincing someone to speak to you. It may be getting support from a consumer health organisation to add 'weight' to your request. It may be making calls to see where there is a bed or room available. It might be finding out how long the waiting list is for a particular operation at different hospitals. It might be doing research online to see what other options are available. It is all about taking a step forward, getting further understanding and then taking another step forward.

Negotiation and mediation often operate closely together, but the specific role of **mediating** is all about getting agreement to a specific course of action. This might be getting agreement to transfer the patient from one hospital to another hospital. It might be getting two specialists to have a phone call to resolve an apparent inconsistency in treatment or medications. It might be getting a new system or procedure implemented for the patient (relating to their meal or access to services). It is an action that achieves a specific outcome for the patient.

To put this all together, a fairly common scenario may start with something like: *"excuse me, but my father has changed his mind and is not comfortable with surgery tomorrow – he has some more questions"* (**interceding**). This may then shift to *"who is the best person for him to speak to? And when would they be available to see my father?"* (**negotiation**) and then conclude by **mediating** to achieve a result: *"OK thank you doctor for making the time to see us again when you are so busy – it's been a tremendous help. Once we can confirm that the rehabilitation program will be OK for dad, and that they have room for him at the centre near my home so I can help him, I think we can proceed with the surgery – that's right isn't it Dad?"*

In each role it is your ability to be assertive, to communicate well, to have empathy and awareness of others and to retain your own 'perspective' (neutrality) that will govern how skilled, effective and 'smooth' you will be in shifting 'gears' between each of these three key roles.

Sometimes you need to use empathy (which in the example above was used in the mediation stage) and other times you need to use assertiveness (by expressing that the patient is no longer comfortable with the surgery). It will be your neutrality and ability to hold your own perspective that will guide you on *how* to approach each role and *when*.

Empathy can be very powerful in interceding, so please do not assume that interceding will always require assertiveness. Expressing statements like *"my mum is just so frightened right now. She won't stop crying. I can hardly imagine how tough this is for her to be facing a cancer diagnosis when her sister passed from cancer last year. I don't think she is quite processing what has been said to her – would you mind coming to see her again? She may not be ready for surgery tomorrow."* This may be much more effective than an approach of *"my mum isn't feeling sufficiently informed to sign the Consent Form. I don't think surgery can happen tomorrow."*

> It is all about using your **neutrality** to weigh up **which role** (negotiate, mediate or intercede) is required, and the **manner** in which that role is best performed (through assertion, empathy, communication, access to knowledge).

In some situations, performing just one of these roles will be sufficient. It might be that once you have **mediated** to bring two specialists or providers together to collaborate more closely for the patient that your work is done! From this point a new treatment pathway may be created and the patient's journey through the health system may be extremely successful. Every case is unique. We simply want you to clearly understand each of these roles so you can feel confident and prepared should you need to suddenly 'engage' and take an action on behalf of your loved one.

MANAGING PACE AND MOMENTUM

Each of the three key roles of a patient advocate: **negotiate**, **mediate** and **intercede**, contains a 'tempo'. A case that requires you to 'intercede' will often have a faster, and more urgent pace to it than a case in which you are mediating or negotiating.

Many of the problems that arise during health care can be attributed to tempo and momentum and therefore not having the time to make clear and informed decisions. If you become aware that you are rushing, or that a faster tempo has entered the situation, you must consciously **STOP** and become aware of the impact this may have upon your own decision-making, the decision-making of health providers and of the patient. Momentum can affect everybody, so this is where you need to use your voice the most to create time and space for good decisions.

If you believe the person you care about is 'slipping through the cracks' of the health system, then you may need to try and **increase** the tempo. If you believe the patient is being rushed into decision-making, then you may need to actively **slow down** the pace or tempo. Taking the time to identify the role that you will be performing will assist you to decide and manage the tempo of your advocacy (and therefore your sense of control) at all times.

A FRAMEWORK FOR PATIENT ADVOCACY

Once you know the patient's preferred outcome and have engaged as positively as you can with the key people who are involved in the patient's health care and treatment, the next step is to develop a strategy for *how* you are going to achieve the result the patient wants.

On the next page is our Framework for Patient Advocacy©. All of the information in this Handbook can be placed into this Framework, and the Framework can be applied to any situation. It will help you to make sure you are in command, have considered all necessary factors and are ready to proceed - *before* you take any action:

A FRAMEWORK FOR PATIENT ADVOCACY©

ISOLATE: Clearly identify the 'core' elements of the situation:

- Who is the patient? (**Who am I helping?**)
- What is the problem? (**What am I here to achieve?**)
- Am I going to: **negotiate, mediate** or **intercede**?
- What is the current 'tempo'? (**Is there momentum?**)

Knowing these 'core' elements (as opposed to focusing on details), is essential to your advocacy being targeted, efficient and effective. This first step of 'isolating' the people, problem and tempo is by far the most important and will govern everything else that you do.

ROTATE: This means examining from all available perspectives:

- the Patient;
- the Problem;
- the Situation (key people, the tempo etc); and
- the Advocate (i.e. You)

Place each of these three elements into the centre of an imaginary 'sphere' and then rotate the sphere to observe that element from as many perspectives as possible. Do you need more information? Are you neutral enough? How is the patient coping?

This step ensures that any stress, confusion or key challenges can be identified and managed from the very beginning.

INTEGRATE: It is essential to 'pause' to consider all of the information that has been obtained to this point. Taking this time will stop any threat from a build in momentum.

PROCEED: Once the steps above have been done, you will be steady, in command and ready to proceed. The 'green light' should not be given to any action until this occurs

HOW TO 'PROCEED'

The issue that is happening will usually show you *how* you should proceed in your advocacy. For example, if a patient's core problem is a lack of communication between the key people involved in their treatment, then your task will be to **negotiate** to arrange some form of meeting or a structure to create collaboration (**mediation**) between those key people – for example by bringing all the key specialists into one room or on one conference call.

In most cases clearly defining the problem or issue, in the context of the patient's 'preferred outcome', will show you the pathway forward. This is why the **Isolate** step is so important.

In Chapter 2 we introduced 'Andrew' who was on a cycle of treatment for his knee. This was a complex case, involving several surgeons and general practitioners as well as numerous medical issues. It was not necessary for the advocate to know at the *beginning* how Andrew's knee could be best managed, only that it was necessary to intercede to prevent Andrew pursuing amputation due to his pain level. The advocate's initial actions were to identify the following:

- That the patient had received 14 procedures, across several different health providers over a period of time;

- That the patient was experiencing daily pain in excess of level '8' on a standard 1-10 pain scale and was taking powerful medication to manage this pain;

- That the patient was desperate and losing the ability to make reasoned decisions;

- That the patient did not appear to be improving under the existing treatment regime;

- That it was necessary to break the treatment cycle to find a new way forward (necessary to intercede);

- That it was necessary to think laterally about accessing new resources (new health providers) to guide the patient forward;

- That it would be necessary for the advocate to be assertive to obtain assistance from these new providers, having regard to the past history; and

- That it would be necessary for the advocate to 'sell' the new approach to the patient to convince the patient not to pursue amputation.

The advocate did not require any prior knowledge to be able to provide effective advocacy services to Andrew. Nor was it necessary to know the final outcome (surgery versus amputation versus physiotherapy) in order to begin. What the advocate *did* require was a framework to guide how they approached the situation. In this case, the advocate applied the Framework for Patient Advocacy in a quick 'summary' format as follows:

ISOLATE:

- Client: Andrew Smith
- Location: Sydney, New South Wales

- Problem: Client wants to end their pain cycle
- Tempo: quite high due to Client's pain
- Role: Intercede to prevent amputation

ROTATE:

- Issues with 'Client':
  - Client has a loyalty to current GP in Sydney;
  - Client is in daily pain;
  - Client is in a state of desperation which is affecting decision making
  - Client's pain level and mobility is not improving
  - Client has lost faith in the system and appears resistant to new strategies

- Issues with 'Problem':
  - Don't know why the Client is experiencing pain;
  - Don't know the source of the pain;
  - Don't know which/if any specific surgery is responsible;
  - Different providers are disagreeing on cause of pain;
  - No provider appears to take any responsibility for pain or finding a solution for Client;
  - Current providers may not be the best sources of a solution

- Issues with 'Advocate':
  - Advocate personally disagrees with amputation as a valid option

> ➢ Advocate does not know what managing constant chronic pain would be like (cannot relate to Client's situation)

INTEGRATE:

- Essential to break the momentum to prevent amputation as this requires ongoing management, including pain management, for Client and thus will not achieve the outcome the Client is really seeking;
- Examine the facts that are known: 14 surgeries have occurred and Client is not improving. Cause of pain is disputed. Unclear if any physical damage exists in knee from surgeries. Lots of uncertainties about matters that should be factually capable of determination (knee is damaged or not damaged, nerves are damaged or not damaged etc). No apparent responsibility or commitment from current providers to address Client's pain.
- Essential to obtain improved factual information as a platform for Client's decision-making.

PROCEED:

- 'Sell' this strategy to Client i.e. worth a try before irreversible surgery that could result in further pain (phantom limb, pain from surgery etc);

- Locate an independent surgeon with good reputation and arrange a consultation for Client as first step in obtaining new factual information; and
- Locate Client's health records for new surgeon to review.

Although this Framework may seem overwhelming, when you break it into steps it becomes quite straight forward. We have used a complicated case to show you that every problem, big or small, can be broken down into manageable steps using this Framework. This is the exact Framework we used to assist Kate and Rose in the example in Chapter 6. This Framework creates safety for you and for the patient because momentum cannot operate when you are applying this Framework. It breaks the cycle and guides your thinking *before* you take any action.

MANAGING 'ROAD BLOCKS'

It is important to recognise road blocks for what they are and not to become frustrated or disheartened if they appear before you during your advocacy. A 'road block' can include not being able to get an appointment, not having phone messages returned by treating providers or receptionists, or being told that a desired treatment option is simply unavailable. Anything that is a 'no' or casts doubt on whether a chosen strategy can succeed is an actual or potential 'road block'.

Your first response when presented with a road block should be to persist with your strategy. It is important not to accept the first 'no', or even the fourth or fifth 'no' that is presented, because the system and the people who are being approached within the system will often be sharing the same pair of 'sunglasses' and may all, initially, believe that 'no' is the correct answer.

If you really believe that a solution can be found and that your strategy is correct, then you should (at least in the short term) keep pursuing the strategy and think of new ways to engage support. Perhaps the patient needs someone else to 'champion' the outcome that is being sought. Perhaps further research is required. Perhaps the communication style being applied is not effective. Perhaps an email will succeed where a phone call will fail. You may need to exhibit stubborn, but respectful, persistence.

If a road block cannot be overcome, then you need to adapt your strategy to navigate around it. This requires the ability to be flexible. Discerning whether flexibility or persistence is required in any given moment is in itself a skill and requires you to use your neutrality to weigh up the success of the strategy to date. If you become personally attached to your strategy you will not be sufficiently objective. You may also take things too personally and start to trigger into your own 'success and failure' cycle which (once again) will affect your neutrality.

Flexibility can also be required if circumstances change and a new strategy needs to be developed. For example, a change in a patient's health situation (for better or worse), can fundamentally change the 'preferred outcome' that you are working to achieve. Being flexible and having the ability to adapt is essential. If the situation has changed then use the Framework again to apply it to the new scenario to help you to review and find a new forward strategy. There is no limit to the number of times you can use the Framework.

Some specific strategies to overcome, or navigate around, road blocks include:

- Changing the situation. Can a new health provider be brought into the decision-making team to lend a fresh perspective?

- Can the patient change where they are being treated? Or receive treatment from another health provider?

- Is there a different or alternative treatment that could be made available to 'break a cycle' and test how the patient may respond?

- Has anyone else experienced the same issue and found a way through?

- Be open to feedback or suggestions from people within the system. If your instinct says that someone is trying to be helpful, listen to their advice. The obstacle may not be as large as you think it is.

- Think about the problem from a completely different perspective in order to see if there is another way forward. It can help to bounce a problem off a friend to try and see it through another 'lens'.

- Work through each of the core qualities of effective patient advocacy to see if a particular skill set has been missed or not optimally applied.

Above all, please do not be too disheartened or discouraged. It is not always possible to move quickly or easily through the health system – these 'road blocks' exist and are very real. This is why it is important to not become too distracted by temporary inconveniences. Keep focused on the 'end game', keep moving forward and keep working to achieve the best result possible in the circumstances.

KEY LEARNINGS FROM CHAPTER 8

- Applying the Framework for Patient Advocacy© will help you to identify the specific actions you need to take to help yourself or someone you care about.
- The first step is to clearly identify the preferred outcome that is sought, as this gives your advocacy focus, clarity and direction.
- You need to know and manage (as best you can) the pace of the health care that is being provided. Health care that is too fast or too slow will cause poor outcomes for the patient.
- Work to engage people to become 'allies' in your advocacy. This requires you to use all the qualities of an effective advocate introduced in Chapter 7.
- It is normal to encounter road blocks or obstacles – what matters is how you respond to these so you can continue working towards the outcome you wish to achieve.

PRACTICE EXERCISE – CHAPTER 8

To help you to become familiar with the Framework we would like you to apply it to one of the Cases from this Handbook or to a situation you are facing.

You may like to use the template provided at the end of this Handbook to assist you.

We have also provided two 'example answers' at the end of this Handbook.

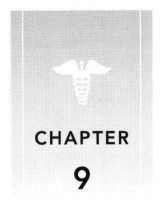

CHAPTER

9

MANAGING DIFFICULT PEOPLE AND DIFFICULT SITUATIONS

Advocacy is fundamentally about engaging with people to achieve an outcome – either for yourself or for someone else. Once you understand the platform for your advocacy and have used the Framework to determine the next course of action, then it is all about implementation – and this will depend upon how effectively you are able to engage with, and manage, other people.

In Chapter 7 we introduced the five core qualities required for patient advocacy. These, combined with the Framework, are the main tools you will need to be able to achieve a result. Sometimes, however, you will encounter people or situations which are especially challenging. This Chapter will therefore provide you with some additional tools to assist you in these more difficult situations so you feel equipped to navigate your way through what you are experiencing.

PREPARE FOR TURBULANCE

You will already have a relationship with the person who is the patient. They could be your friend, partner, child, parent or colleague. This relationship will have all the natural complexities and dynamics that exist in all interpersonal relationships. When this relationship changes to one in which you are also their advocate and they are the patient (and are consequently feeling unwell, frightened and/or in pain) then this relationship will obviously become even more complicated!

The patient may be experiencing trauma and be unable to communicate with you. Or they may express anger or rudeness towards you that is upsetting and unreasonable. They may blame you or resent you. They may suddenly feel uncomfortable about you knowing their medical information. There are all kinds of complexities that can develop in the context of providing patient advocacy and so it takes skill and awareness on your part to navigate all the dimensions of your relationship with the patient while they are receiving care. The more prepared you are for these complexities the better you will be able to manage them!

KNOW YOUR TRIGGERS

Neutrality is your greatest ally in patient advocacy. It is what will keep you clear-sighted, focused and *stable* no matter what is happening in your relationship with the patient. The **Rotate** step in the Framework is all about helping you to maintain this neutrality, as much as is possible, in the circumstances you are facing.

To give you an example, **Rotate** is what will support you to see that you are upset at the moment because your sister (who is the patient) is refusing to speak with you. It will also help you to see that the reason your sister is upset is because she just got a bad test result. So rather than reverting to a childhood pattern of sibling 'wounding', the best thing for you to do is just to sit quietly by her bed while she processes the information and be ready to support her to think about the next action to take when she is ready. But, if you can't see beyond your own pain and the 'unfairness' of her reaction, you will not be stable and ready to help her when she needs it.

This is why you need to have some self-awareness and know your own 'personal triggers' as much as you can.

> You need to make *conscious* the feelings, desires and reactions that may be *unconscious* and then manage the situation accordingly. Remain focused on the patient and the outcome you are trying to achieve and know that there will be plenty of time for you to process your own feelings and reactions later on.

Maintaining neutrality also means knowing some of *your* personal characteristics that could cause issues for *other* people. For example, some people have a natural confidence that others can mistake for arrogance. Their 'default' position is that they know best, and the other person does not. People such as this rarely say 'sorry' and genuinely mean it. At the other end of this spectrum are people who 'can never get it right'. They believe all problems are their fault. They say 'sorry' for everything and can suffer from low self-confidence and low self-worth. If you were to have a cup of coffee with either of these 'people', it is likely that at some point you would get irritated!

This is why it is so important to look in the mirror at yourself if any relationship problems arise, as you may have contributed to what is occurring. This could be conscious or unconscious. You may be tired, stressed and not as tolerant as you usually are. Or you may be feeling frightened for the patient and be losing your own stability. If anything like this happens (which is natural and normal) then just steady yourself, regain your neutrality and take steps to get the relationship back on track.

PATIENTS WHO ARE 'CHALLENGING'

It is very easy for the person who is the patient to jeopardise a health outcome that they actually wish to obtain. This will rarely be deliberate. Because you already know the person, it is likely you will also know what the person is like and how they are likely to behave, but you may not be prepared for this in the context of a health issue. The following is a guide to help you to manage these situations.

People who are emotional and/or dramatic

Some people are highly emotional and/or dramatic. They may see the very worst in every possibility, may cry extensively, may be highly sensitive, may feel depressed and refuse to speak and may want everything to be attended to 'as an emergency'. They may also want a lot of your time and attention.

People who are highly emotional can be exhausting to manage due to their inherent lack of perspective. They see only their own needs and own situation and nothing else. They do not see any other point of view so they will not see what you are trying to do for them – they will only see the situation in relation to themselves.

Your neutrality will help you to manage through this, because their behaviour is exactly why they need an advocate! Health providers are likely to find the person difficult to deal with, so their treatment could be subtly impacted by their behaviour. This is why you are needed, so try not to take the behaviour personally and focus on getting the best result you can. By focusing on the 'end game' you will reduce the chance that everyone (including the patient) will remain distracted by the 'daily dramas'.

Patients who are in trauma and/or unclear
or inconsistent in their instructions

A patient may be unable to provide you with clear and consistent instructions and information. They may be experiencing trauma and be in a state of shock, they may continually change their mind, or they may have an inherent misunderstanding or belief around their condition that makes it difficult for you to help them.

In these situations, you first should try and obtain information direct from the patient's medical team (with the patient's permission) to confirm the situation and the options available. You may then be able to 're-set' the patient about what is occurring and reduce the confusion that they may be experiencing.

If they are experiencing trauma or are in shock, you will need to exercise special care. People who are in trauma often need to feel there is plenty of time and space for them to absorb and process what is occurring. Rushing people in trauma or overloading them with too much information will create the opposite outcome to what you intend. The best support you can provide may be to remove any unnecessary stimulation, pressure or distractions and assist the patient to have their basic physical and emotional needs met. This may be ensuring they are warm, have adequate food and water, are able to watch a familiar television show as well as locating a social worker, counsellor or psychologist if necessary to provide specific support and assistance.

If the patient is frequently changing their mind, you should try and work out why this is occurring. Are they receiving pressure or being influenced by someone else? Are they nervous about committing to a course of action? Are they frightened? It is important not to dismiss patients who are like this as being silly, because they may simply be trying to please everyone – including you – and may have lost track of their own desires and wishes. Using empathy to build trust may assist them to speak honestly with you and to commit to a course of treatment.

Patients who are 'experts'

The Internet has made a large amount of complex medical information highly accessible. This information is also available in books, magazines and from 'friends who are doctors'. It is very common for people to conduct their own medical research and to engage in 'self-diagnosis'. This is a serious challenge for medical practitioners and health providers.

This is also a mechanism some people use to feel more empowered in their health care and treatment. At the same time, the reliability of the information, the relevance of it to the specific patient as well as their ability to properly comprehend complex medical information and language can be very questionable.

It is always best to encourage any patient who is uncertain about the information they have received to obtain a second (or even a third) opinion and be extremely cautious about pursuing any strategies that have been formed through self-diagnosis.

THE PATIENT ADVOCATE HANDBOOK

Patients who are 'dishonest'

It can be very difficult to help a patient who is dishonest with you or with their health team. They may drink or be smokers but not wish to tell their health providers. They may lie about symptoms they are or are not experiencing or about whether or not they have complied with a health plan previously provided to them.

Once again this is where you need to use your neutrality and empathy to attempt to understand *why* the person is being dishonest. Are they frightened? If so, reassure them and assist them to become more honest with their health team. If the person prefers, you can inform the health team for them and save them any embarrassment. Remember it is a key responsibility for patients in health care that they are honest and open with their health team in order to create safe and efficient health outcomes.

Patients who aren't ready to become healthy

Some patients, particularly patients who have suffered with a health condition for a long period of time, can become heavily invested in their health issue and may in fact build their identity around being unwell or suffering from a particular ailment or condition. Most of the time the patient will be completely unaware that this is occurring. This type of situation will manifest through a general reluctance by the patient to explore new treatments. They will be subconsciously *working against* you finding a solution to their health issue.

Ultimately it is up to the patient to decide what outcome they want. It is not for you to decide what is best for them. If the patient is not yet ready to move towards a solution, then there is little you can do. The responsibility once again lies with the patient.

MANAGING 'DIFFICULT' PEOPLE

Sometimes the people involved in the patient's health care and treatment will be difficult to work with and so you will need to exercise extra skill to navigate *around* them to achieve the health outcome you are seeking.

Managing People Who Are Rude, Angry and/or Aggressive

It is possible that you will encounter people who are rude, angry and/or aggressive towards you at some point. This behaviour may range from a general lack of respect and courtesy, to an arrogant disregard, to walking away from conversations, to swearing and shouting or worse.

It is natural to be hurt, offended or even to feel frightened when presented with behaviour of this kind. This behaviour is not appropriate and is unacceptable. However, it can occur, and so you need to be prepared for how you will respond if it is ever directed towards you.

As much as possible try and remain calm, in command of yourself and focus upon how you can reduce the intensity of the interaction. Although it can be tempting to 'talk back' to the person concerned, this will rarely achieve anything other than to escalate the conflict. Make sure that everyone is safe from physical harm. If you are at all worried about your physical safety walk away and, if necessary, get help. At no point and under no circumstances should you be exposed to physical danger.

Assuming there is no risk to physical safety, the next step is to maintain, or if necessary, regain, your neutrality. **Rotate** and consider *why* the person is behaving in this manner. Is it their natural (if misguided) way of asserting their power? Are they feeling threatened? Are they frightened? Are they sleep-deprived and stressed? What is *behind* the display of emotional behaviour that is being presented?

It is not uncommon for people to experience anger when they feel a loss of control. This can easily happen when expectations are not being met. It is your neutrality that will enable you to have perspective. The more that you can identify what the 'real issue' is, the more opportunity you will have to resolve it. Using empathy as a technique to diffuse the tension and create a 'bond' can be successful – this can even convert someone who was 'difficult' into an ally.

If the person is a health provider, then if all of your attempts to work with the person have failed, you should consider whether you can by-pass the person. Can the patient be transferred to another practitioner? Can a Patient Representative at the hospital be consulted? Can a formal complaint be lodged against the person? Patients will understandably be anxious that any direct action will have an adverse consequence on their health care, and so you will need to make sure that the patient is reassured and agrees before taking any steps of this kind.

Managing People Who Are Obstructive

You may encounter people, especially people who work within the health system, who appear (to you) to be obstructive. This means that they are not willing to engage or cooperate with you to develop or find a new solution to the patient's situation.

If you become aware that a person is obstructive, then you must reconsider your strategy immediately, as you may only have one chance to get the relevant person 'on board'. This is why communication is such an important quality of an effective advocate, as you must be able to listen as well as to speak. You need to be aware of how your approach to any person who has a position of power is being received, and be flexible enough to change your approach – mid-sentence if necessary!

When people appear to be obstructive, empathy will generally be more effective in achieving a solution than assertiveness. This is because the person concerned is likely to be comfortable with their power and in how they exercise it. The key to a solution will be in convincing the person that they *want* to help you and the patient, and this will have the greatest chance of succeeding through the use of empathy.

If you believe the person is acting inappropriately then once again you may need to consider whether a Patient Representative can help, or if a formal complaint should be lodged to obtain a forward movement for the patient.

MANAGING DIFFICULT SITUATIONS

Different people will find different situations to be 'difficult', but any situation in which someone you love is in a potentially life-threatening position is obviously very stressful.

Bad News

It is always hard for a patient to receive 'bad news', and this is especially the case when the bad news is unexpected. 'Bad news' can range from receiving a diagnosis that has an uncertain future (for example, there are treatments available but no guarantee that they will be successful), to the news that a serious surgery must occur for the patient to recover, to the worst possible news that the situation is terminal and there is nothing more that can be done.

Because of your relationship with the patient, both you and the patient are likely to suffer from shock and be distressed – and you both may require support and assistance. It is unreasonable to expect that you will be neutral and stable at this time – just do the best you can.

We recommend that you try and get a trusted third party involved at this point to provide advocacy support to you and to the patient. At times like this it will be very hard for you to remain an 'advocate' when you are also 'a daughter'.

You may wish to pass this Handbook to the new support person so they can read about the Framework and can work with you and the patient to formulate a new strategy. If the future actions are not yet clear, it can help to break a case into 'stages' so everyone can see that there is 'a plan' and feel more empowered within that plan.

Depending on the situation, the patient may require help in other areas such as in managing employment-related issues and leave entitlements, accessing superannuation, accessing home support services (especially meals and cleaning support), booking pets into a kennel or cattery, organising a power of attorney or similar so someone can pay the patient's bills and manage their affairs, and so on.

When There is No Hope

It is extremely distressing for patients and people close to the patient to hear that nothing further can be done and that the patient is not going to recover from what they are facing. There will be shock, fear and disbelief. Everyone involved becomes faced with their own mortality and their own experience of loss.

In these situations it is once again essential that a trusted third party is brought in to provide advocacy and personal support. The patient needs someone to assist them who can maintain some neutrality and, due to your personal relationship with the patient, you will find this very difficult if not impossible. This is perfectly normal – you are not letting anyone down! In fact, bringing someone in to help and be a stabilising influence may be the most responsible course of action for you to take.

When it comes to answering the question 'how much time do I have?' many health providers wait to be guided by the patient as to what they want to know. Some patients want to know, while others may not be ready to deal with this and need time to come to terms with the reality of their situation before knowing their 'timeframe'.

It can be difficult for health providers to deliver this news as their focus is to 'do and cure'. Not all providers are sensitive to the impact of their news, and in their own personal discomfort may appear to be 'cool' towards the patient's situation and not give them sufficient time to digest the information. If you, or the new support person, are present, it is important to be aware that this can occur, not to take it too personally and to support the patient to obtain all the information they need when ready. This may require scheduling an additional appointment in a few days' time to enable the patient to absorb what they have been told and to prepare a list of questions.

Whoever is now performing the role of patient advocate is there to assist the patient to understand the diagnosis, to support them if they want to explore and access other treatment options and to refocus on what can be done to help the patient be more comfortable to the greatest extent possible. Throughout this whole process, the patient, the family (and you) may also need support in accessing grief counselling.

Emergency situations

We have provided some support on how to handle emergency situations in Chapter 1. The most important thing is to remain as calm as possible and to prevent momentum from taking hold. If you are able to apply the Framework this will also help you to maintain clarity and focus.

KEY LEARNINGS FROM CHAPTER 9

- Your existing relationship dynamics with the person who is the patient are likely to become more complicated while they are receiving health care.
- The more you can prepare yourself for this extra complexity in your personal relationship, the more you will be able to manage it.
- Neutrality and the ability to apply the Framework to 'Rotate' to see other people's points of view will help you to maintain clarity and perspective so you can remain focused on the work to be achieved.
- Some people and situations are especially difficult to navigate and require additional preparation, skill and support to handle effectively.

CHAPTER

10

CARING FOR THE PATIENT ADVOCATE

Sometimes being able to help someone you love in a practical and meaningful way can really help you to manage your own stress and trauma about their health issue. You at least know that you are doing all you can to help them towards the best possible health outcome that is available.

At the same time, it is very important to manage and look after yourself because you can only be as effective as your personal 'reserves' will allow. It is impossible to care for someone else if you are unable to care for yourself. This Chapter will therefore focus on practical ways you can manage and look after yourself while being a patient advocate for someone you love and care about.

MANAGING YOUR INITIAL EMOTIONAL RESPONSE

It is natural to be emotionally impacted by what you are seeing, experiencing and handling. Someone you care about is undergoing a significant health issue and health issues are always stressful because they can be so unpredictable. You are not a robot, and you should not make your emotions wrong. You are allowed to feel angry, sad, upset, scared and overwhelmed. This is normal and perfectly fine.

If you are in the middle of a situation and something happens which upsets or stresses you, then you need to try to regain your equilibrium as much as you can so you can handle what is happening for the patient in this moment. It is possible that your own 'flight or fight' response may trigger, which means you will suddenly be charged with adrenaline and may also become quite unsteady.

It is important to recognise when you have lost your stability and to do what you can to calm yourself down. You will be able to take time and process how you feel later, but someone may be relying on you right now so you need to do the best that you can to stabilise. Here are some simple techniques which may assist you:

- Remove yourself from the situation, even if only for a few moments, so you can regroup. The toilets can be very useful for this, however going outside and getting some fresh air is ideal.

- Stay calm. You may have been shouted at, blamed for a bad outcome or been present when bad news was delivered. Whatever has occurred, it is essential to breathe and to calm down. You will be of no value to anyone if you are upset.

- Take the intensity out of the situation, including out of your own reaction and emotions. Let the impact of what you feel pass through you and let it go as much as you can for the time being.

- Use visualisations. Imagine yourself being 'bullet proof' or with a force field so you can try and protect yourself from what is happening.

- Have something to eat. Sometimes eating can help you to feel nurtured. Forget calories – eat what makes you feel calm!

- Use humour. You may say something funny to yourself. Say or do something that helps you to distract yourself so you can regain your balance and refocus on the task at hand.

- Remind yourself that all that matters is achieving the result. How the patient or how health providers feel about you in this moment is not as important as the work you are doing. Respect comes from the outcomes you achieve and the manner in which you achieve them.

- Remember that the situation is extremely frightening and traumatic for the patient as well. You are in this together.

- Seek support if you need it. This may be from a professional, family or friends.

These techniques are not long-term solutions. They are only to help you to stabilise so you can help the person who is the patient – they need you!

MANAGING INFORMATION

The health system is often described as a world of its own with its own rules, customs and language. If you are not familiar with the terms that are used (including some very long words!) you can find the information quite overwhelming. You may even feel silly or stupid if you cannot pronounce or understand key words.

We recommend that you start taking notes as soon as you can of as much detail as you can. This could be in a notepad or on your phone or iPad. Keep track of medications, dosages, allergies, the frequency of pain, any changes that are made to treatment, the names and contact details for key doctors, the ward, specialists, and so on.

Doing this will help you to achieve three important outcomes: first, it will be very helpful for the patient's medical team as they will be able to check key facts with you, and you will also be alert to any changes or mistakes. Second, it will help free your mind from overload as you won't need to remember every detail. You will be able to simply refer to your notes whenever information or historical data is needed. Finally, it will help you to feel more in command, as slowly you will become familiar with the language and key terms used.

MANAGING YOUR PERSONAL 'LOAD'

Most people lead busy lives and have a lot of 'balls in the air' at the same time. They might have young children. They might be caring for an elderly parent. They might run their own business. They might be renovating their kitchen. They might be doing all of these at the same time! And then a health issue comes along and suddenly they are also a patient advocate.

It is easy to become overloaded, because a lot of people do not maintain 'contingencies' in their lives – they tend to fill their lives and their time and so there is often little capacity to manage unexpected, protracted and stressful events.

An approach we have found very useful is to see each person as always having 100 'Units' of energy available to allocate as they see fit. This includes Units that are necessary for sleep/ rest, for eating, for spending time with family, for conducting activities (including work, study or other activities), for recreation and so on.

Each person must allocate their Units in the way that is best for them. Sometimes there is a lot of choice in how this allocation occurs, and at other times there is less choice. People who are unwell, for example, have less choice because their body will suddenly require them to allocate a lot of Units to resting and recuperation. This does not mean the other areas of their life suddenly require less Units – it is just that they don't have the Units available to spread across all the areas of their life in the way that they did before they became unwell.

It is the same for you. You only have 100 Units available. Of these 100 Units, you will need to decide how many Units should be applied to each area of your life, including the advocacy work you are now doing. No matter how talented at multi-tasking you are, there will come a point where you start to become overloaded. When this happens, it is important to know that you have simply run out of Units.

It is common when people start to run out of Units that they increasingly operate from adrenaline. Part of them knows that they are heading into danger and so their natural 'fight or flight' instinct can trigger, and the adrenaline can make them feel that they can handle more than they really can. In addition to making it harder to **Isolate, Rotate** and **Integrate** to make considered decisions, at some point the adrenaline will run out and the person will 'crash'. It is far better, in the long term, to operate at a more balanced and sustainable pace. Running on adrenaline can easily turn into letting momentum run you!

When you start to run out of Units there are four key strategies you can use to help you to re-set and stabilise:

Learn to Say 'No'

It is essential that you start to say 'no' to everything that you can say no to. You may not be able to go to dinner with friends. You may not be able to take on an extra client or project at work. You may not be able to attend a school function. This will not be the situation forever – but right now while you are doing this advocacy work you simply don't have any Units to spare and each one of these activities requires Units. Learn to say 'no' until you have the Units available to say 'yes'.

Plug the Leaks

There may be people, situations or activities in your life that drain you. When you have enough Units you can handle these elements, but when you run out of Units you simply cannot afford them.

Leakages are situations or people who take more from you than they should. It can feel like your 'life force' or sense of wellbeing is falling away and for no real outcome. It might be a neighbour or friend who wants to make small talk or complain endlessly about something that cannot be changed. It might be waiting in a queue for 20 minutes for a meal. It can be anything that requires Units that you simply don't have available for that person or situation.

You need to protect every single Unit of energy you have by 'plugging the leaks' – because each Unit is too precious to waste. Be as polite as you can be, but actively avoid situations and people who are 'leaks' for you at the moment. Make conscious decisions about where you eat, how you travel and what you do so you manage yourself well. It might be slightly more expensive to catch a taxi or an Uber to get from Point A to Point B, but it won't drain you as much as travelling on a busy train.

Re-Allocate Your Units

If at all possible, consciously reallocate how you use your Units – and delay or let go of anything that can be delayed or removed. If you are about to renovate your kitchen see if you can push it back a month to when you will have the Units available to handle it. Use time in this way to create space for yourself – because if you have a breakdown, it will all have to be delayed anyway!

There may be commitments you have agreed to, classes you have signed up for, decisions you have made. Everything should be reassessed in light of what is now happening for you. No one benefits from you collapsing, and people understand that health crises occur. It is important not to think you can continue as you did before you started being an advocate. You need to adapt to what is *actually* happening. Put as much as you can 'on hold' and only handle the essentials.

Accept Imperfection

The final technique is perhaps the most important. If you are reading this Handbook then you are someone who likes to do things well. You may even be a perfectionist. Unfortunately, perfection has to go out the window when health issues occur, and it is impossible to manage everything the way you usually do when you run out of Units. There will always be something you miss: paying a bill, meeting a friend, spending time with your child, making a phone call.

The sooner you can make peace with imperfection, the healthier and calmer you will become. Life happens. Everything will stabilise at some point – between now and then you just need to relax, let go of perfection and do the best you can. If you were helping a friend who was trying to handle all that you are handling, you would probably counsel them to do the same thing. Take the pressure off yourself, know you are doing your best and accept life as it is for the time being.

BUILD YOUR RESILIENCE

Helping someone during a health challenge can be exhausting. There are hours spent waiting for information, results or appointments. There are often no answers. Everyone around the patient is busy and under various levels of stress and pressure. It's no picnic! This is why in addition to managing your Units you also need to learn how to build your personal resilience so you can 'go the distance' while remaining as neutral and stable as you can throughout the journey.

Know It Is Not Personal

Although at times the reaction, opposition or resistance you experience may *feel* very personal, you need to *know* that it is not personal. People are just busy and if you are (in their eyes) slowing them down or making their job harder by asking for more information or more time, then they may express and direct frustration towards you.

It is not personal. Most people just like doing their work in the way that they like to do it, especially if they are under pressure. So 'shake it off' as best you can. It is also important that you do not subtly start to seek their approval or avoid asking questions because of their reaction. Your neutrality is essential for you to remain focused and on course – no matter how they feel about you!

Recognise Your Motivation

Why are you doing what you are doing? What is your motivation? Is it love? Is it responsibility? Are you the only person who can do this? It can really help you to remember *why* you are helping the person you are helping. There is always a motivation, and this 'personal truth' is what will help you the most when you are encountering opposition and resistance. It is what will give you the strength, conviction and courage necessary to say 'no', to keep going and to push against resistance for the outcome you are seeking.

Take Regular Breaks

It is essential to take frequent, short breaks whenever you can. Ideally, go outside and get some fresh air. Take a short walk. Breathe and try to calm your nervous system because the tension of health care will be causing all sorts of subtle (and not so subtle) stresses for you. Having short breaks allows to you to clear your mind so you can remain focused.

If you cannot leave the building, take short walks around the ward to give yourself a break from the intensity and constancy of being 'on alert'. If you don't find small ways to look after yourself it will be difficult for you to go the distance.

Get Support

Finally, talking to someone about how you are really feeling can be a wonderful tonic. It might be a friend, a relative or a professional – what matters is that you can express yourself and what you are experiencing. Having a sounding board and getting feedback and support can be of enormous help. Do not feel that you are being weak or needy taking this step – it may be essential!

MANAGE YOUR GUILT

Just because you are providing advocacy support to someone you care about does not mean you are an expert or that you are responsible for what happens to them. **A bad outcome can happen despite your very best efforts.**

If the patient's health journey does not go as planned, it is natural for you to feel responsible and to experience guilt. This is normal. You have taken on a lead role (you have been driving the car!) and you didn't get to the right destination. This can be an awful feeling, but it is not your fault. You have not done anything wrong. Health is unpredictable, and you cannot control whether someone has a good or a bad test result. All you can do is try and make their journey through the health system as safe and steady as possible.

> You may need to be very strong with yourself at this point and really tell yourself the truth: **you have done the best you can, and you are not responsible for their health result**. Keep telling yourself this because it is the truth.

It may be necessary for you to speak with a professional to 'debrief' what has happened. You may feel confused, disempowered, angry and guilty – all at the same time. If you don't express what you are feeling and get support, then these emotions will build up within you and cause negative outcomes in other parts of your life.

The reason health issues are traumatic is because we have such little control, so please don't let the role of patient advocate confuse you into believing you have control over health – this is never the case! All a patient advocate can ever do is try and improve the process of health care by managing momentum, empowering the patient to make good decisions and being by their side throughout the journey.

KEY LEARNINGS FROM CHAPTER 10

- To be effective as an advocate for someone else you need to look after yourself. This means learning how to manage your own emotional experience around what is happening, managing your 'workload' and building your resilience.
- It is not your fault if the person you are helping has a negative health outcome. You are not responsible. All you can do is try and make the process of their health care as safe and effective for them as possible. You cannot control their actual health.
- It is essential to get support (including professional support) to help you to process and understand what you have been through and experienced as a patient advocate.

PRACTICE EXERCISE – CHAPTER 10

Write down all the key commitments, focuses and activities in your life right now. Then allocate 'Units' to each of these commitments, focuses and activities (the total number of Units must equal 100). Include sleep, exercise, socialising, work – everything.

The purpose of this Exercise is to help you to become aware of your current 'load', so you can make conscious decisions to create capacity as early as you can *before* running out of Units and experiencing the stress and issues that this creates.

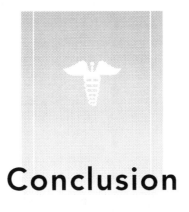

Conclusion

In this Handbook we have brought together all we have learned to assist you to build confidence and belief in your capacity to help yourself or someone you love while experiencing a health challenge.

Health issues are extremely stressful, tiring and unpredictable. By using the Framework for Patient Advocacy© you will be able to remain focused and strategic each step of the way.

The main keys to remember are as follows:

- Use the Framework as much as possible – it will keep you focused.

- The enemy of good decision-making is momentum. Manage the tempo (don't let it manage you!)

- You will need to either negotiate, mediate or intercede to create a result.

- Your neutrality will help you to know which role to perform and when.

- Your neutrality will also help you to know whether you should use empathy or assertiveness as your primary approach when seeking to achieve an outcome.

- Look after yourself as much as you can along the way.

- Above all – your voice is your greatest asset, so learn how to use it effectively!

Interested in learning more?

For additional tools, checklists and resources please visit our website:

www.thepatientadvocatehandbook.com

We wish you every success in your journey through the health system.

APPENDIX 1

PRACTICE EXERCISES (SAMPLE ANSWERS)

CHAPTER 2

Case Study: Mary (Mediate)

Sample answers are as follows:

- The dominant action in this case was to mediate between Mary, her husband and the hospital staff. This was needed to resolve the conflict and distress caused by Mary's medical condition and the dislocation arising from her treatment. The patient advocate was able to create an environment where both sides were made aware of the others' concerns (Mary's isolation from her family against the hospital's desire to ensure that Mary was receiving appropriate care) and a resolution was achieved.

- A range of parties were involved in this case and the family were not being heard in relation to the struggles they were experiencing due to Mary being admitted to a hospital located far away from her regional home. A new common ground was mediated between Mary, her family, the treating team and metropolitan hospital.

- The dominant action taken by the patient advocate was b) to mediate. There were entrenched issues that needed to be resolved to create an opening that would allow for a solution that would support Mary and her family. The family addressed the hospital's concerns and found a regional hospital that would provide appropriate rehabilitation. This allayed the hospital's concerns that Mary would not receive the care she needed and they then felt clear to support her being transferred to a facility closer to home.

Case Study: Andrew (Intercede)

Sample answers are as follows:

- In this situation the Patient Advocate was engaged by Andrew to see if there was an alternative to a fairly drastic surgical procedure, above knee amputation. The Patient Advocate studied Andrew's case history and decided on seeking an independent review of the case. This resulted in Andrew changing his providers which ultimately resulted in him seeking alternative treatment with good results. This is a clear case of interceding in the flow of an existing health care treatment but at the request of the patient.

- Intercede- The flow of health care involved further surgery and potential amputation of Andrew's leg. Interceding as an active intervention was necessary to create a 'wedge' in the flow of health care - this was done by seeking a second opinion and recommendation for an alternate treatment strategy which involved physiotherapy and delay of further surgery.

- The dominant action taken by the patient advocate was c) to intercede. In this situation the patient advocate created a wedge in the flow of health care being provided which had been a cycle of continual surgical operations. This was the catalyst for Andrew receiving independent advice which started him working with a new team on a radically different treatment strategy. The intervention changed the direction of his treatment.

Case Study: Daniel (Negotiate)

Sample answers are as follows:

- The Patient Advocate was able to facilitate, through negotiation with the relevant personnel, a smoother and speedier admission and treatment process for Daniel.

- The Patient Advocate negotiated with the hospital to determine if a better solution could be found to address the issue of Daniel's health worsening when he was forced to wait in the Emergency Room for treatment.

- Negotiate - Daniel was experiencing negative outcomes due to long waits in the emergency department during acute exacerbations of his illness. Negotiation occurred with the treating team and hospital to initiate a new intake procedure on Daniel's presentation to hospital that facilitated admission and immediate treatment.

- The dominant action taken by the patient advocate was a) to negotiate. The patient advocate negotiated with the specialist, campaigned with the hospital and facilitated collaboration between the two to establish a new in-take procedure to enable Daniel to receive treatment on admission.

CHAPTER 3

Case Study: Jessica (Sample Answer 1) - Respect

Let us say that Jessica is extremely deaf without her hearing aids. She is also very anxious about being in hospital, asking lots of questions, and she is sometimes forgetful, which means she doesn't always remember what she has asked or been told. Respecting Jessica's right to be fully informed about her health care would present some challenges. Among strategies which could be used would be:

- Ensuring that Jessica always has her hearing aids on or within easy reach, with the batteries fully charged;
- Wherever possible, speaking to Jessica in an area where there is not a lot of background or incidental noise so she has a better chance of understanding what is being said;
- Recognising that her hearing loss means communicating with her may take a little longer than with someone with excellent hearing;
- Suggesting that Jessica keeps a day book or similar where she can write down questions she wants to ask and then record the answers; and
- Recognising her anxiety and being ready to spend a few extra minutes to explain what is happening and to ensure that Jessica has understood the explanation.

Case Study: Jessica (Sample Answer 2) - Participation

Personalised as follows: Jessica is awaiting heart surgery following a history of high blood pressure. Jessica has been advised one possible complication from surgery is a significant risk of stroke. She has been a long term smoker. She lives alone and enjoys a full and engaging life. Life in a Nursing

Homes is not an option for her in the future, if she has a say in it.

1. Jessica discloses her fear that she will have a stoke during the surgery and become disabled and need nursing home care. She is explicit she would not want this. The health professional advises her about the opportunity to make an Advanced Care Directive, which she does with her designated support person being vested with medical power of attorney to implement this directive.
2. The Surgeon and anaesthetist would inform her about the options for her health care, the consequences of each option, using non-medical language, diagrams and physical models demonstrating the procedure. She would be encouraged to ask questions with her support person in attendance.
3. Jessica would be given time to consider her option and as much information as she required to provide informed consent when signing the Consent to Treatment form. Her fears would be acknowledged and not diminished by any health care workers.
4. Jessica would be advised that she has the right to refuse treatment of change her mind and withdraw consent to treatment. Her health care workers would support her choice and not retaliate in a negative way if she declined a treatment option or changes her mind.
5. Jessica's is consulted on the optional procedures for heart surgery and she is present and involved in decision making about her care, in both medical and surgical consultations, while in hospital.
6. Jessica has received information and it has been presented to her in a language she can understand and at a level of health literacy that she is comfortable with.

7. Jessica has the opportunity to consult family about proposed treatments and delay treatment in order to consult her family, her GP or designated support person.
8. Jessica has a right to say what outcomes she is looking for from the treatment and these outcomes should be translated into a patient centred goal, i.e. Jessica wants to be able to walk down to the shops and remain independent living and attend her clubs and cultural group.
9. Jessica will be invited to attend her medical team review post operatively and any adverse outcomes will be openly reported to her under the open disclosure policy of the health service
10. Jessica will be advised of her rights if she has a complaint about her care and referred to complaints and advocacy groups re any concerns without negative repercussions.

Case Study: Jessica (Sample Answer 3) - Respect

Jessica is 70 years old - not suffering from Dementia and not deaf and has lived with her female Partner for over 20 years so:

- Including Jessica on any decisions relating to her healthcare

- speak normal volume (Not speaking loudly) to her when Nursing staff take observations;

- Allowing Jessica to make her own decisions relating to dietary requirements and ancillary health care;

- Allowing Jessica Complimentary Therapists (Homeopaths / Masseurs to make a hospital visit);

- Discuss openly with Jessica and any of her nominated caring staff results of tests already undertaken and procedures being considered;

- Simply allowing her visitors to attend during a procedure she finds confronting and stressful understanding that they must not hinder the procedure in any way;

- Informing Jessica's partner of the current situation and including her partner in any discussions relating to Jessica's healthcare; and

- Allowing Jessica to shower herself privately and visit the toilet without intervention given that she is fully able bodied and capable without risking her health further.

CHAPTER 4

Case Study: Stan

Guided by the Australian Charter of Health Rights, Stan has a right to actively participate in his treatment plan and should be supported to seek the second (or third) opinion he is requesting. In addition, he should be supported to access a support person or formal advocate of his choosing. Given Stan does not have a mobile phone with him, the hospital should provide practical support via creating access to a phone for him to use.

The Charter is not legally enforceable - however there are common law rights that can be applied.

In Queensland Stan has the right to refuse medical treatment if he is deemed to have the capacity to understand the implications of treatment and refusing treatment- without providing consent the surgeon is unable to remove the hand.

The Surgeon has an obligation to provide Stan with information about the treatment including outcomes, risks, side effects, alternate options and financial considerations. In this case he owns a business has a mortgage, business loan and overdraft. Loss of his hand will have severe financial implications; hence this needs to be discussed with him by the surgeon.

Stan is able to seek the second opinion, but he may be liable for the out of pocket costs. Medicare does not place a restriction on the number of second opinions that can be sought - the challenge is if the surgeon or the GP refuse to make this referral. In this case Medicare does not pay the rebate. A concern for Stan is that he may be unable to leave the hospital; therefore access to a second opinion of his choice will be restricted - for example his choice of surgeon may be limited or he may have to pay private consultant fees.

If the hospital and surgeon are unhelpful and do not support Stan to seek a second opinion, he is able to lodge a complaint at the hospital or with the Health and Quality Complaints Commission about the care he is receiving.

This does not appear to be an emergency situation where an exception to the rule for consent may apply (for example if he was unconscious and removal of the hand would save his immediate life).

In Stan's case he may not die as a result of his refusal to have surgery-but a high level of alternate care and treatments will be required to try to 'save' the hand. In this situation the surgeon has a right to refuse to treat the patient if they are of the belief that treatment is futile.

If he was assessed not to have the capacity to consent the surgeon needs to determine if Stan has: appointed an Enduring Power of Attorney, has an Advanced Health Directive, or has a statutory health attorney. If these are not in place a substitute decision maker can be appointed. In this case it is his sister who lives overseas would be the first nominee for this role as he is not married (assume he does not have defacto). If they are not able to access the sister, or the next closest relative that he has a relationship with then they could apply to the Queensland Civil and Administrative Tribunal (QCAT) for consent

CHAPTER 8

Case Study: Kate (Chapter 6)

Isolate –

- Client – Kate
- Location – Kalgoorlie
- Problem – Management of treatment for patient, Rose
- Role – Negotiate with hospital re Rose's pain management on behalf of Client

Rotate –

- Issues with Client

    o Client is exhausted and distressed and fearful of what might happen both to the patient and to herself
    o Patient has ongoing pain coupled with withdrawal symptoms and need for ongoing surgery
    o Patient is distressed and traumatised by her experiences with the hospital system to date

- Issues with Problem

  - o Unclear if current drug regime is causing patient's psychosis but has definitely caused adverse allergic reaction
  - o Hospital is assessing drugs but still thinks it's the best program for the patient
  - o Client has alternative remedy, but it is a strong opiate and addictive

- Issues with Advocate

  - o Advocate does not know what managing constant chronic pain or caring for a child in these circumstances would be like
  - o Advocate has concerns about giving a 12-year old ongoing doses of opiate

Integrate –

- Essential to break momentum and delay Rose's discharge from hospital overnight to give Client time to have a break and recover her equilibrium
- Examine the facts as known. The current drug regime is having adverse side effects (possibly psychosis and definitely allergic reaction). The solution proposed by the Client is opposed by the doctors because of the potential for addiction. There is no acknowledgement by the hospital that Rose is a danger to herself and to her mother and that the Client does not have the ability to manage another psychotic episode or allergic reaction (such as if Rose stops breathing again).
- Essential to obtain better factual information so the Client (together with Rose, if she is capable) can make an informed decision on how to proceed.

Proceed –

- Discuss strategy with the Client;
- Negotiate with hospital to keep Rose overnight;
- Locate an independent specialist with a good reputation in pain management and arrange a consultation
- Locate Rose's health records for the new specialist to review

Case Study: Jessica (from Chapter 3) – with hypothetical facts

Isolate –

- Client: Jessica Smith (patient)
- Location: Adelaide, South Australia
- Problem: Client wants to ensure full recovery from Hip Replacement
- Role: Negotiate in the best interests of the client and their health

Rotate –

- Client Issues

    o Client has bias against health providers and staff and is constantly suspicious of their intentions
    o Client has lost faith in the system after many years of impaired movement and lack of choices as to how to address
    o Client finds it difficult to stop and rest
    o Client is in defacto relationship which is not recognised and is concerned for Partner's involvement should their opinion be sought

- Problem Issues

  o Lack of trust by the patient of the system is becoming debilitating and impacting on health of client
  o Partner's influence on the client is impacting on client's ability to relax and focus on their recovery
  o Rehabilitation programme difficult to enact without Partners involvement (to a large degree).

- Advocate Issues

  o Advocate would like client (patient) to be able to speak more independently from their perspective (rather than through the partner)
  o Advocate personally sees some level of independence is healthy and encouraging responsibility of ones actions
  o Advocate does not know whether decision being made in relation to rehabilitation is suiting the client or the Partner.

Integrate –

- Essential to establish client's goals post-surgery e.g. (regain full movement and independence)
- Essential to meet with both Client and partner and discuss openly goals and roles in the process in regaining "full recovery" and what that means

Proceed –

- Locate a local to client Physiotherapist and Lifestyle Coordinator who will develop a rehab programme that will suit and work for Client.
- Meet with the surgeon and client and discuss options and likely decisions to be made throughout operation and post-operative period. Lay out plan of who then is in best position to make those decisions at the time on behalf of the client e.g. Surgeon, partner, client.
- Meet with the allocated Anaesthetist and the client and partner and discuss risks associated, any preferred anaesthetics and actions by the partner should issues ensue.
- Research hip replacement process independently to be better informed for the client. Speak with known colleagues who have undergone this procedure to gain their insights and suggestions as to best practices for recovery.

APPENDIX 2

A FRAMEWORK FOR PATIENT ADVOCACY©

(This Template may be copied for your personal use only)

STEP 1: ISOLATE

Who is the patient? (**Who am I helping?**)

_____

What is the problem? (**What am I here to achieve?**)

_____

_____

_____

Am I going to: **negotiate**, **mediate** or **intercede**? Why?

_____

_____

What is the current 'tempo'? **(Is there momentum?)**

_____

_____

STEP 2: ROTATE

Are there any issues, complications or 'hot spots' with the Patient?

_____

_____

Are there any issues, complications or 'hot spots' with the Problem?

_____

_____

Are there any issues, complications or 'hot spots' with the Situation (Key people, health providers, the tempo? Etc)

_____

_____

Are there any issues, complications or 'hot spots' within you or for you?

_____

_____

STEP 3: INTEGRATE

Stop and reflect. What is really happening here? What is causing poor outcomes? Does the tempo need to be changed (sped up or slowed down)? Is your initial preferred role of negotiate/mediate/intercede still appropriate? What additional information is required? Can the problem be broken down into separate stages which can be handled one at a time? Write your thoughts.

_____

_____

_____

_____

STEP 4: PROCEED

You should now be able to identify your next step. It might be obtaining a second opinion; arranging a meeting of specialists; it might be consenting to surgery; it might be going home. There should be one clear 'next step' that emerges once you have completed the preceding three Steps. Once this is identified you can give the 'green light' and proceed to take the action written below:

_____

_____

_____

If the situation should change, or if you should meet a 'road block' or obstacle, please complete the Framework again to identify the best way forward in the circumstances. There is no limit to the number of times you can use this Framework for any problem or crisis you are facing.

END NOTES

CHAPTER 2

1   For example please refer to the American Hospitals Association < http://www.aha.org > See also *Readings: 'The Patient's Bill of Rights: AHA* < http://www.qcc.cuny.edu/socialsciences/ppecorino/ MEDICAL ETHICS TEXT/Chapter 6 Patient Rights/Readings The%20Patient Bill of Rights.htm >

CHAPTER 3

2   Kerridge, I, Lowe, M & Stewart, C *Ethics And Law For The Health Professions,* The Federation Press, (4th ed.) Sydney 2013, 1046. See also White, B et al Health Law in Australia Lawbook Co, (3rd ed.) Sydney 2018, 123.

3   United Nations. *International Convention on Economic, Social and Cultural Rights* Geneva, United Nations, 1966. Article 12, see < http:// www.ohchr.org/EN/ProfessionalInterest/Pages/CESCR.aspx >, see also White, B et al Health Law in Australia Lawbook Co, (3rd ed.) Sydney 2018, 123-125.

4   Office of the United Nations High Commissioner for Human Rights and the World Health Organisation, *The Right To Health - Fact Sheet No.31, S. B, 5,* see < http://www.humanrights.gov.au/right-health > and < https://www.ohchr.org/Documents/Publications/Factsheet31. pdf >

5   Office of the United Nations High Commissioner for Human Rights and the World Health Organisation, *The Right To Health - Fact Sheet No.31, S. B, 5,* see < https://www.ohchr.org/Documents/Publications/ Factsheet31.pdf >

6   See for example Australian Human Rights Commission, Human Rights Explained Fact Sheet 5: The International Bill of Rights, see < https://www.humanrights.gov.au/our-work/education/human-rights-explained-fact-sheet-5the-international-bill-rights >

7   Australian Commission on Safety and Quality in Health Care, *Australian Charter of Healthcare Rights,* Sydney NSW < http://www.safetyandquality.gov.au/national-priorities/charter-of-healthcare-rights/ >. Most states and territories in Australia have adopted their own version of the Charter. For more information please see White, B et al Health Law in Australia Lawbook Co, (3rd ed.) Sydney 2018, 103-105.

8   Australian Commission on Safety and Quality in Health Care, *Australian Charter of Healthcare Rights,* Sydney NSW < http://www.safetyandquality.gov.au/national-priorities/charter-of-healthcare-rights/ >

9   Australian Commission on Safety and Quality in Health Care, *Australian Charter of Healthcare Rights,* Sydney NSW < http://www.safetyandquality.gov.au/national-priorities/charter-of-healthcare-rights/ >

10 The following information is derived from the Australian Commission on Safety and Quality in Health Care, *Australian Charter of Healthcare Rights,* Sydney NSW < http://www.safetyandquality.gov.au/national-priorities/charter-of-healthcare-rights/ >, this information is primarily derived from Department of Health, State Government of South Australia, *Your Rights and Responsibilities – A Charter for Consumers of the South Australian Public Health System,* June 2012 < http://www.sahealth.sa.gov.au/wps/wcm/connect/Public+Content/SA+Health+Internet/Health+topics/Legal+matters/Your+rights+and+responsibilities >; Department of Health, State Government of Victoria, *The Australian Charter of Healthcare Rights in Victoria,* May 2011 < http://www.health.vic.gov.au/patientcharter/ >; Department of Health, State Government of NSW, *Your Health Care Rights and Responsibilities,* < https://www.health.nsw.gov.au/patientconcerns/Pages/your-health-rights-responsibilities.aspx >

CHAPTER 4

11 See for example White, B et al Health Law in Australia Lawbook Co, (3rd ed.) Sydney 2018, 136-138.

12 *Schloendorff v The Secretary of the New York Hospital* 211 NY 125 (1914) at 129-130, which was applied in Australia in *Secretary, Department of Health and Community Services (NT) v JWB and SMB (Marion's Case)* (1992) 175 CLR 218 at 233.

13 *Rogers v Whitaker* (1992) 175 CLR 479 at 489.

14 United Nations. *International Convention on Economic, Social and Cultural Rights* Geneva, United Nations, 1966. Article 12, see < http://www.ohchr.org/EN/ProfessionalInterest/Pages/CESCR.aspx > and see for example *Charter of Human Rights and Responsibilities Act 2006* (VIC) http://www8.austlii.edu.au/cgi-bin/viewdb/au/legis/vic/consol_act/cohrara2006433/ section 10(c).

15 White, B et al Health Law in Australia Lawbook Co, (3rd ed.) Sydney 2018, 140-141.

16 White, B et al Health Law in Australia Lawbook Co, (3rd ed.) Sydney 2018, 141.

17 White, B et al Health Law in Australia Lawbook Co, (3rd ed.) Sydney 2018, 148. See also Kerridge, I, Lowe, M & Stewart, C *Ethics And Law For The Health Professions,* The Federation Press, (4th ed.) Sydney 2013, 344.

18 White, B et al Health Law in Australia Lawbook Co, (3rd ed.) Sydney 2018, 145-147.

19 *Re T (Adult: Refusal of Treatment)* [1993] Fam 95 at 113, per Lord Donaldson.

20 See Kerridge, I, Lowe, M & Stewart, C *Ethics And Law For The Health Professions,* The Federation Press, (4th ed.) Sydney 2013; White, B et al Health Law in Australia Lawbook Co, (3rd ed.) Sydney 2018; *Rogers v Whitaker* (1992) 175 CLR 479.

21 *Rogers v Whitaker* (1992) 175 CLR 479. See also Kerridge, I, Lowe, M & Stewart, C *Ethics And Law For The Health Professions,* The Federation Press, (4th ed.) Sydney 2013, 357.

22 *Rogers v Whitaker* (1992) 175 CLR 479. See also Kerridge, I, Lowe, M & Stewart, C *Ethics And Law For The Health Professions,* The Federation Press, (4th ed.) Sydney 2013, 357.

23 *Rogers v Whitaker* (1992) 175 CLR 479; *Chappel v Hart* (1998) 195 CLR 232.

24 *Chappel v Hart* (1998) 195 CLR 232 at [10].

25 See Kerridge, I, Lowe, M & Stewart, C *Ethics And Law For The Health Professions,* The Federation Press, (4th ed.) Sydney 2013, 365. See also White, B et al Health Law in Australia Lawbook Co, (3rd ed.) Sydney 2018, 140.

26 *Hunter and New England Area Health Service v A* (2009) 74 NSWLR 88 at [28]. See also White, B et al Health Law in Australia Lawbook Co, (3rd ed.) Sydney 2018, 577.

27 See for example *Medical Treatment Planning and Decisions Act 2016 (Vic)* < http://classic.austlii.edu.au/au/legis/vic/num_act/mtpada201669o2016397/ > section 58(2).

28 *Re T (Adult: Refusal of Treatment)* [1993] Fam 95 at 102; see also See also White, B et al Health Law in Australia Lawbook Co, (3rd ed.) Sydney 2018, 577 and Kerridge, I, Lowe, M & Stewart, C *Ethics And Law For The Health Professions,* The Federation Press, (4th ed.) Sydney 2013, 350.

29 *Re T (Adult: Refusal of Treatment)* [1993] Fam 95 at 113. See further *Medical Treatment Planning and Decisions Act 2016 (Vic)* < http://classic.austlii.edu.au/au/legis/vic/num_act/mtpada201669o2016397/ >; White, B et al Health Law in Australia Lawbook Co, (3rd ed.) Sydney 2018 and Kerridge, I, Lowe, M & Stewart, C *Ethics And Law For The Health Professions,* The Federation Press, (4th ed.) Sydney 2013.

30 *Re B (Adult: Refusal of Medical Treatment)* [2002] 2 All ER 449; *HE v A Hospital NHS Trust* [2003] 2 FLR 408 at 414; Re T *(Adult: Refusal of Treatment)* [1993] Fam 95 at 102; see also White, B et al Health Law in Australia Lawbook Co, (3rd ed.) Sydney 2018, 143-150.

31 See for example the *Medical Treatment Planning and Decisions Act 2016 (Vic)* < http://classic.austlii.edu.au/au/legis/vic/num_act/mtpada201669o2016397/ > section 3. See also *Gardner; re BWV* [2003] VSC 173; *Bridgewater Care Group (Inc) v Rossiter* [2009] WASC 229.

32 See White, B et al Health Law in Australia Lawbook Co, (3rd ed.) Sydney 2018, 217-218.

33 See White, B et al Health Law in Australia Lawbook Co, (3rd ed.) Sydney 2018, 218.

34 See White, B et al Health Law in Australia Lawbook Co, (3rd ed.) Sydney 2018, 218.

35 See White, B et al Health Law in Australia Lawbook Co, (3rd ed.) Sydney 2018, 219-220.

36 See for example Kerridge, I, Lowe, M & Stewart, C *Ethics And Law For The Health Professions,* The Federation Press, (4th ed.) Sydney 2013, 400-401.

37 See White, B et al Health Law in Australia Lawbook Co, (3rd ed.) Sydney 2018, 220-227.

38 See White, B et al Health Law in Australia Lawbook Co, (3rd ed.) Sydney 2018, 154-155.

39 See White, B et al Health Law in Australia Lawbook Co, (3rd ed.) Sydney 2018, 141-145.

40 *Re C (Adult: Refusal of Medical Treatment)* [1994] 1 WLR 290; see also White, B et al Health Law in Australia Lawbook Co, (3rd ed.) Sydney 2018.

41 Kerridge, I, Lowe, M & Stewart, C *Ethics And Law For The Health Professions,* The Federation Press, (4th ed.) Sydney 2013, 642-646, White, B et al Health Law in Australia Lawbook Co, (3rd ed.) Sydney 2018; see also as an example World Health Organization Aging and Life Course < https://www.who.int/ageing/ageism/en/ >

42 Kerridge, I, Lowe, M & Stewart, C *Ethics And Law For The Health Professions,* The Federation Press, (4th ed.) Sydney 2013, 642-646, White, B et al Health Law in Australia Lawbook Co, (3rd ed.) Sydney 2018; see also as an example World Health Organization Aging and Life Course < https://www.who.int/ageing/ageism/en/ >

43 Kerridge, I, Lowe, M & Stewart, C *Ethics And Law For The Health Professions,* The Federation Press, (4th ed.) Sydney 2013, 589.

44 *Gillick v West Norfolk and Wisbech AHA* [1986] AC 112 at 189, which has been applied in Australia in *Secretary, Department of Health and Community Services (NT) v JWB and SMB (Marion's Case)* (1992) 175 CLR 218.

45 See Australian Medical Association Code of Ethics (Revised 2016) cl 2.2.2 at < https://ama.com.au/position-statement/code-ethics-2004-editorially-revised-2006-revised-2016 >, I, Lowe, M & Stewart, C *Ethics And Law For The Health Professions,* The Federation Press, (4th ed.) Sydney 2013, 298-300. See also White, B et al Health Law in Australia Lawbook Co, (3rd ed.) Sydney 2018, 397-398.

46 *Hippocratic Oath*, as translated by the United States' National Library of Medicine < http://www.nlm.nih.gov/hmd/greek/greek_oath.html >

47   Office of the Australian Information Commissioner, *Australian Privacy Principles* < http://www.oaic.gov.au > and see also < https://www. oaic.gov.au/individuals/my-health-record/about-my-health-record >

48   See for example *Varipatis v Almario* [2013] NSWCA 76.

CHAPTER 5

49   Merriam-Webster Online Dictionary, *Culture* < http://www.merriam-webster.com/dictionary/culture >

50   Business Dictionary.Com, Values < http://www.businessdictionary. com/definition/values.html#ixzz2eow7NaNK >

51   Merriam-Webster Online Dictionary, *Morality* < https://www.merriam-webster.com/dictionary/morality >

52   For example the Crimes Act 1900 (NSW), Division 12, Sections 82-84 < http://www.austlii.edu.au/au/legis/nsw/consol_act/ca190082/ >

53   World Health Organization, Regional Office for Europe, Weight bias and obesity stigma: considerations for the WHO European Region, see < http://www.euro.who.int/_data/assets/pdf_file/0017/351026/ WeightBias.pdf >; see also Senderovich, H *How Can We Balance Ethics and Law When Treating Smokers?* Rambam Maimonides Medical Journal (2016) Apr. 7(2) see < https://www.ncbi.nlm.nih.gov/ pmc/articles/PMC4839538/ >

54   Medical News Today, *40% of Medical Students Unconsciously Biased Against Obese People* < http://www.medicalnewstoday.com/ articles/260967.php >

55   Merriam Webster Learners Dictionary < http://www.learnersdictionary. com/definition/neutrality >

56   Merriam Webster Online, Neutrality < http://www.merriam-webster. com/dictionary/neutrality >

57 Merriam Webster Online, Neutrality < http://www.merriam-webster.com/dictionary/neutrality >

CHAPTER 7

58 Encyclopedia Britannica, *Empathy, 245-248,* 1999, accessed online from< https://www.britannica.com/science/empathy >

59 See for example von Devivere, B *Meaningful Work: Viktor Frankl's Legacy for the 21st Century*, Springer 2018 at 120.

60 See for example Zaki J, *Using Empathy to Use People: Emotional Intelligence and Manipulation*, Scientific American (2013, November 7) < https://blogs.scientificamerican.com/moral-universe/using-empathy-to-use-people-emotional-intelligence-and-manipulation/ >

61 See for example Duffy, J *Empathy, Neutrality and Emotional Intelligence: A Balancing Act for the Emotional Einstein* QUT Law Review, Vol 10 No 1 (2010) < https://lr.law.qut.edu.au/article/view/9 >

62 See for example: Barratt, C, 'How To Show Empathy', *Maxwell School of Citizenship And Public Affairs,* 2006.

63 Oxford Online Dictionary, *Communication* < http://oxforddictionaries.com/definition/english/communication >

64 Windle, R and Warren S, *Communication Skills*, see < https://www.cadreworks.org/resources/communication-skills > (please note: we have used this reference extensively in this Chapter as we find it very simple and practical to apply). See also < https://www.habitsforwellbeing.com/9-effective-communication-skills/ >

65 Windle, R and Warren S, *Communication Skills*, see < https://www.cadreworks.org/resources/communication-skills >

66 Windle, R and Warren S, *Communication Skills*, see < https://www.cadreworks.org/resources/communication-skills >

67 Windle, R and Warren S, *Communication Skills*, see < https://www.cadreworks.org/resources/communication-skills >; please see also

< https://www.skillsyouneed.com/ips/nonverbal-communication.
html >

68 Windle, R and Warren S, *Communication Skills*, see < https://www.
cadreworks.org/resources/communication-skills >

69 Windle, R and Warren S, *Communication Skills*, see < https://www.
cadreworks.org/resources/communication-skills >

70 Windle, R and Warren S, *Communication Skills*, see < https://www.
cadreworks.org/resources/communication-skills >. See also Katz, N,
& McNulty, K, Reflective Listening, *Maxwell School of Citizenship And
Public Affairs, 1994,* < https://www.maxwell.syr.edu/uploadedFiles/
parcc/cmc/Reflective%20Listening%20NK.pdf>

71 Windle, R and Warren S, *Communication Skills*, see < https://www.
cadreworks.org/resources/communication-skills >; see also Tygani,
B *Listening: An Important Skill and its Various Aspects* The Criterion
Issue 12, February 2013 < http://www.the-criterion.com/V4/n1/Babita.
pdf >

72 Windle, R and Warren S, *Communication Skills*, see < https://www.
cadreworks.org/resources/communication-skills >; see also Tygani,
B *Listening: An Important Skill and its Various Aspects* The Criterion
Issue 12, February 2013 < http://www.the-criterion.com/V4/n1/Babita.
pdf >

73 Windle, R and Warren S, *Communication Skills*, see < https://www.
cadreworks.org/resources/communication-skills >

74 To learn more please see for example *4 Types of Communication
Styles*, Posted March 27, 2018, Alverina University < https://online.
alvernia.edu/articles/4-types-communication-styles/ >

75 The following is based on Katz, N, & McNulty, K, Reflective Listening,
Maxwell School of Citizenship And Public Affairs, 1994, < https://
www.maxwell.syr.edu/uploadedFiles/parcc/cmc/Reflective%20
Listening%20NK.pdf > (please note: we have used this reference
extensively in this section as it is available online and is very clear
and helpful). Please see also Riddle, J, *5 Things To Practice For*

Effective Communication, January, 20th, 2013 < http://workawesome. com/communication/effective-communication-skills/ >

76 Katz, N, & McNulty, K, Reflective Listening, *Maxwell School of Citizenship And Public Affairs, 1994,* < https://www.maxwell.syr.edu/ uploadedFiles/parcc/cmc/Reflective%20Listening%20NK.pdf >

77 Katz, N, & McNulty, K, Reflective Listening, *Maxwell School of Citizenship And Public Affairs, 1994,* < https://www.maxwell.syr.edu/ uploadedFiles/parcc/cmc/Reflective%20Listening%20NK.pdf >

78 The following techniques have been derived from Katz, N, & McNulty, K, Reflective Listening, *Maxwell School of Citizenship And Public Affairs, 1994,* < https://www.maxwell.syr.edu/uploadedFiles/parcc/ cmc/Reflective%20Listening%20NK.pdf >

79 The 7C's of Communication are attributed to Cutlip, S and Center, A (1952) *Effective Public Relations: Pathways to Public Favor.* See also Executive Education, *The Seven Cs of Communication,* 28th June 2017 < https://edexec.co.uk/the-seven-cs-of-communication/ > and Mulder, P 7 C's of Effective Communication (2012) accessed via ToolsHero < https://www.toolshero.com/communication-skills/7cs-of-effective-communication/ >

80 The 7C's of Communication is attributed to Cutlip, S and Center, A (1952) *Effective Public Relations: Pathways to Public Favor.* See also Executive Education, *The Seven Cs of Communication,* 28th June 2017 < https://edexec.co.uk/the-seven-cs-of-communication/ > and Mulder, P 7 C's of Effective Communication (2012) accessed via ToolsHero < https://www.toolshero.com/communication-skills/7cs-of-effective-communication/ >

Printed in the United States
By Bookmasters